ARTIFICIAL INTELLIGENCE IN DENTISTRY

A MANUAL FOR FUTURE DENTISTRY

DR. SWARNAA CHATURVEDI

Copyright © Dr. Swarnaa Chaturvedi
All Rights Reserved.

This book has been published with all efforts taken to make the material error-free after the consent of the author. However, the author and the publisher do not assume and hereby disclaim any liability to any party for any loss, damage, or disruption caused by errors or omissions, whether such errors or omissions result from negligence, accident, or any other cause.

While every effort has been made to avoid any mistake or omission, this publication is being sold on the condition and understanding that neither the author nor the publishers or printers would be liable in any manner to any person by reason of any mistake or omission in this publication or for any action taken or omitted to be taken or advice rendered or accepted on the basis of this work. For any defect in printing or binding the publishers will be liable only to replace the defective copy by another copy of this work then available.

To 'the epitome of strength and my support system - **my mother**, *'the man of principle and my source of encouragement -* **my father**, *'the purest soul on this planet, my inspiration, and my Santa' -* **my brother** *and 'the one full of zeal and my unconditional twin friend' -* **my sister.**

Contents

Preface

Artificial Intelligence is a burgeoning segment with its branches extending into every sphere, and dentistry is not an exception. However, its concepts are arduous to understand and are not yet compiled as one source from the point of view of dentistry. This fact made me frame a book on the application of AI in dentistry and present my readers with literature having intelligible language and tabulated details.

This book covers almost all the notable studies about the application of AI in dentistry conducted so far. This book can be used by budding dental undergraduates, postgraduates as well as clinicians to bring these models into practical application. In addition, this could also be used by AI professionals who wish to put their skills in the realm of dentistry.

I have put all the possible efforts into providing readers with correct information. However, being human beings, mistakes are inevitable. Therefore, I request my readers to inform me about any mistakes if found.

I hope to bring revolution in the field of dentistry through this book, and even if I could plant the seed of applying AI into dentistry in only a few minds and bridge the gap between the great minds of dental professionals and AI professionals, that would do justice to my hard work that I have put in this book.

Dr. Swarnaa Chaturvedi

Acknowledgements

"NO ONE WHO ACHIEVES SUCCESS DOES SO WITHOUT THE HELP OF OTHERS. THE WISE AND CONFIDENT ACKNOWLEDGE THIS HELP WITH GRATITUDE."

– Alfred North Whitehead

The words are few, and language seems feeble when the heart is full of gratitude.

Words cannot express my deep sense of gratitude and respect to my mentors, **Dr. Priya Singh, Dr. Neeta Misra, Dr. Deepak U., Dr. Saurabh Srivastava, and Dr. Puja Rai**, their logical suggestions and meticulous attention to detail, which has helped me bring this work to its ultimate goal.

Words cannot describe my emotions toward my beloved parents, **Mr. A. C. Chaturvedi and Mrs. V. L. Chaturvedi,** and my elder sibling **Dr. Apoorva C.**, without their constant inspiration, unconditional love, and support, I might not be the person I am today and lots of love to my loving sister **Mrs. Kavya C.**, whose smiling face is the premier stress buster for me.

I would like to thank my colleagues and friends, **Dr. Himanshi, Dr. Mona, Dr. Sarah, Dr. Ribhu, Dr. Priyanka, and Dr. Gaurav**, for their valuable support and suggestions whenever needed them.

And last but not least 'I thank **Lord Krishna**, the merciful and the passionate, for giving me the strength to keep going.

Dr. SWARNAA CHATURVEDI

CHAPTER ONE

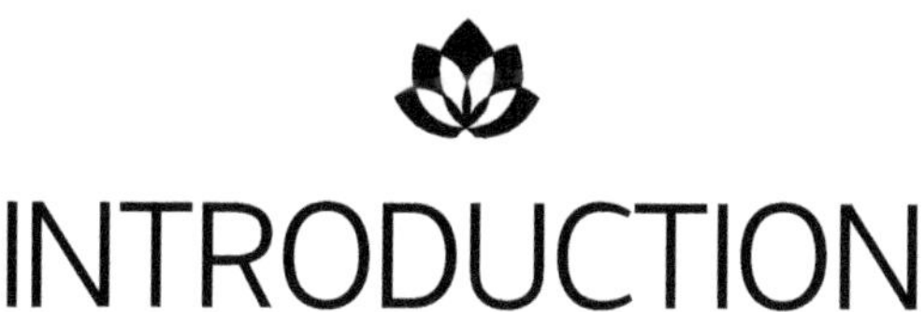

INTRODUCTION

"Artificial intelligence is almost a humanities discipline. It's really an attempt to understand human intelligence and human cognition."
-Sebastian Thrun

1.1 Background

Human Intelligence is unique among this variety of intelligence because of its unparalleled ability to design, modify and build new forms of intelligence. Human intelligence is what defines us as humans and our relationship with everything on earth. While in no case can artificial intelligence replace the role of a dental surgeon but it is important to be acquainted with the scope to amalgamate this advancement of technology in the future for the betterment of dental practice.

Artificial intelligence (AI) is a budding field yet considerably established in the medical and dental fields. Algorithms, mathematical calculations, computerized data collection methods, and an enormous amount of reproducible data are the basis of machine learning, a subcategory of AI that is helping to improve areas of dental care in ways once unimaginable. From the basic step of taking a patient's history to data processing and then extracting the information from the data for diagnosis, artificial intelligence has many applications in dental and medical science. (1) Hence, there is a requirement for dentists to understand its potential implications for a remunerative clinical practice in the future. (2)

AI was first coined by John McCarthy and refers to machines that can imitate human knowledge and behavior. (3)

1.2 Frequently Used Definitions

1.2.1 Classical Definitions:

The classical definitions of artificial intelligence are organized into four categories broadly for purpose of better understanding (4)

? Thinking Humanly
"The automation of activities that we associate with human thinking, activities such as decision-making, problem-solving and learning." (Bellman, 1978)
"The exciting new effort to make computers think... machines with minds, in the full and literal sense." (Haugeland, 1985)

? Thinking Rationally
"The study of mental faculties through the use of computational models." (CharniakandMcDermott,1985)
"The study of the computations that make it possible to perceive, reason, and act." (Winston,1992)

? Acting Humanly
"The art of creating machines that perform functions that require intelligence when performed by people." (Kurzweil, 1990)
"The study of how to make computers do things at which, at the moment, people are better." (Richand Knight,1991)

? Acting Rationally
"Computational Intelligence is the study of the design of intelligent agents." (Poole et al.,1998)
"AI is concerned with intelligent behavior in artifacts." (Nilsson,1998)

1.2.2 Other definitions:

AI is defined as a field of science and engineering concerned with the computational understanding of what is commonly called intelligent behavior and with the creation of artifacts that exhibit such behavior. (5)

According to "Barr and Feigenbaum," AI is the part of computer science concerned with designing an intelligent computer system that exhibits characteristics we associate with intelligence in human behavior-understanding language, learning, reasoning, problem-solving, and many more. (5,6)

In 1978 Richard Bellman, an applied mathematician, defined artificial intelligence as the automation of activities associated with human thinking abilities, which includes learning, decision making, and problem-solving. In the modern-day world, artificial intelligence refers to any machine or technology that is able to mimic human cognitive skills like problem-solving. To understand AI, it is important to know a few of these key aspects. (7)

Artificial intelligence (AI) is defined as the study of intelligent agents, any device that perceives its environment and takes action that maximizes its chance of successfully achieving its goals (Russell and Norvig 2003) (4)

When the term "AI" was introduced, it meant a system that was operated in the same way as human intelligence through non-natural, artificial hardware, and software construction, meaning strong AI. The concept of strong AI first requires an adjustment of the definition of intelligence. Here, intelligence is defined as "the capacity of a system that can act appropriately in an uncertain environment."(8)

Weak AI means a system in which human beings take advantage of some medical and logical mechanisms in which intelligence works to efficiently execute intellectual activities that a human can perform. (9)

1.3 Model of AI

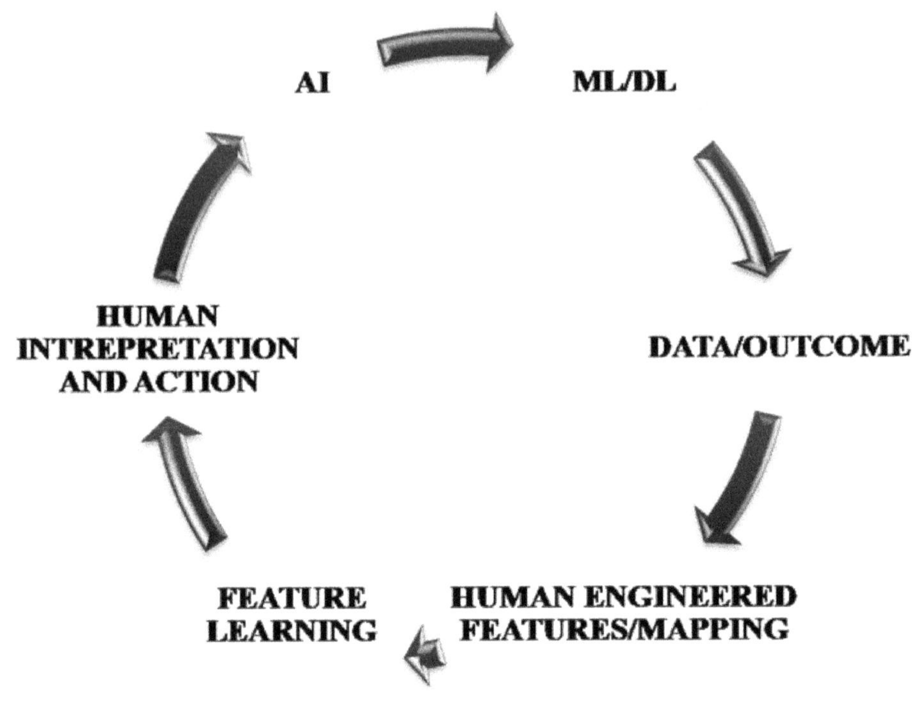

Figure 1. Showing standard model of working of AI(10)

1.4 Branches of AI

Branches of ARTIFICIAL INTELLIGENCE can be broadly grouped as (4)

a. ROBOTICS
b. NEURAL NETWORKS
c. EXPERT SYSTEMS
d. NATURAL LANGUAGE PROCESSING
e. FUZZY LOGIC
f. MACHINE LEARNING

1.5 Types of AI

Artificial intelligence can be of two forms:
1. Weak
2. Strong

Weak Artificial Intelligence

Its use in medical and logical mechanisms might be advantageous to human beings to perform intellectual activities with the help of intelligence neural networks. (11)

The concept of weak AI intends to improve the cognitive behavior and judgmental capacity of computer systems to make them inherent in those computing systems, denying the unreasonable reduction and in an attempt to reproduce the human intelligence, which is predicted and planned by strong intelligence. (12)

Strong Artificial Intelligence

It is a scheme that works similarly to human intelligence through the construction of some unnatural software and artificial hardware. It is the capacity of the machine to swiftly and efficiently perform and reproduce human behavior with prime features including communication, learning, planning, puzzle-solving, making a judgment, and reasoning ability. (13)

1.6 Terminologies

Common terminologies used in artificial intelligence (5,14,15)

1.6.1 Machine learning (ML)

Machine learning was first discussed by Arthur Samuel in 1959. (1) Machine learning is a component of artificial intelligence that depends upon the protocol to generate results supported by data sets. A sub-type of machine learning is representation learning, in which the categorization of data is done from the algorithm systems generated by computers. The only difference between Machine Learning and Representation learning is that there is no need for hand-labeled data, which is required in machine learning. (12)

Machine learning constitutes the algorithm strained to perform tasks by learning patterns from data rather than by explicit programming. Therefore, machine learning techniques invariably involve parameter tuning with regard to the underlying technique. (16)For example:

? Number of neurons, layers, and epochs in a neural network technique
? Membership functions election in fuzzy logic.
? Population size, selection strategy, mutation rate, and cross-over rate in genetic algorithms, as well as in the hybrid techniques that use fuzzy logic or neural network, or both.

1.6.2 Representation learning

It is a subtype of Machine Learning in which the computer algorithm learns the features required to classify the provided data and does not require hand-labeled data like ML.

1.6.3 Deep learning (DL)

Another sub-type is "deep learning, which utilizes varied computational layers through a deep neural network, thus analyzing the input data. The goal is to generate patterns to improve feature detection."
DL is an aspect of AI which refers to artificial neural networks (ANN) with complex multilayers.

Deep learning has more complex ways of connecting layers and also has more neurons count than other networks to express compound models. As a result, it possesses more computing power to train and further has automatic extraction of the feature.

This algorithm uses multiple layers to detect simple features like lines to complex shapes, lesions, or whole organs in a hierarchical structure.

1.6.4 Clinical decision-support systems (CDSS)

Almost everyone born in this century has tons of medical and genetic information documented in some way or the other. A lot of this information may not be relevant, but now as more and more links are being identified between genes and susceptibility to dental diseases, the process of finding any relevant genetic information, although tedious, may prove to be an irreplaceable insight into the accurate diagnosis and treatment of dental diseases.

A Clinical decision support system (CDSS) can perform this function quite efficiently. A Clinical decision support system (CDSS) is a network between an extensive dynamic (medical) knowledge database and an inferencing output mechanism that is a set of algorithms derived from evidence-based medical practice implemented through medical logic modules such as Arden syntax. (17,18,19)

Most CDSS has four essential components:

1. Inference Engine(IE)
2. Knowledge Base (KB)
3. Working Memory
4. Explanation Module

1. Inference Engine (IE) - It is the central part of any such system which contains the knowledge about the patient from which certain conditions can be concluded.

2. Knowledge Base (KB) - The knowledge used by IE is created to facilitate the acquisition and elicitation of this knowledge.

3. Working memory –It is a message stored in a database having collected patient data.

4. Explanation Module – It is not present in all CDSS. It is responsible for composing justifications for the conclusions drawn by the IE in applying the knowledge in the KB against patient data in working memory.

Another system that is used to predict genetic disorders and susceptibility to the same is the genetic algorithm (GA), which is a search heuristic that mimics the process of natural evolution. (20) Up until the last decade, the most tedious part of this process was to enter structured information into the system, but with the advent of voice recognition and the ability of artificial intelligence programs to identify and extract information from scanned paperwork, this process has been simplified. (4) Added to this is the interactive inter-phase that is designed to assist the health care professional in comprehending vast amounts of information more efficiently than human assistants and simultaneously bridge the gap between the doctor and the patient. These interactive interphase assist the health care professionals in working more efficiently with a time-saving and cost-effective clinical dental practice. (18,21)

1.6.5 Artificial neural networks (ANNS)

ANN is a highly interconnected network of computer processors that are inspired by the biological nervous systems. Mc Culloch and Pitts invented the first artificial neuron in IN1943.(12,22,23) Later, Frank Rosenblatt, a psychologist, developed the Perceptron in 1958, which worked on a multilayer feed-forward mechanism. Another breakthrough came when Paul Werbos, in 1974, instigated "backpropagation" learning.

Currently, this feature of computer programs is being used to "grab" newer information and aid the health industry with data processing and knowledge representation. Multiple layers of computer processors capable of performing parallel computations for data processing make up these networks. Each of these units is known as "neurons," and they are interconnected by links, each of which has a numerical weight associated with it.

ANN consists of artificial neurons or nodes connected in hierarchical layers:

An input layer-> One or more hidden layers -> An output layer

Each node, except for the input neurons, receives multiple weighted inputs followed by producing output that is usually a nonlinear function of the inputs. Their ability to learn from historical examples, analyze nonlinear data, handle imprecise information and generalize, enabling the application of the model to independent data, has made them a very excellent analytical tool in medicine.

For example, they have been used in:
o Clinical diagnosis
o Image analysis in radiology
o Histo pathology

Data interpretation in the intensive care setting and waveform analysis. These systems help connect dental healthcare professionals all over the world. (24)

With their personal smart devices, the patients can enter the symptoms they are experiencing and be conscious of the most probable diagnosis of the illness. Today there are mobile applications available that help patients identify malignant melanomas by comparing the pictures from the patient with avast interphase pictures of lesions from around the world. (eg. Mole Check App, Online Derm Clinic, Skin XM). (25) A similar system can be applied and implemented for the self-examination of suspected oral cancerous lesions. This technology helps patients to get an expert opinion at the earliest while also helping dental health care professionals to prioritize the appointments when necessary.

A study done by Kim et al. used an Artificial neural network to build a model that can predict toothache on the basis of the association between toothache and daily tooth brushing frequency, tooth brushing time, use of dental floss, toothbrush replacement pattern, oral hygiene maintenance, dental checkups and other factors like diet and exercise. This successful study aided the development of a toothache predictive model with great accuracy. This model recognizes adequate eating habits, oral hygiene, and stress prevention as the most important factors in preventing toothaches.

Another research used Bayesian network analysis to identify relationships between various factors affecting the diagnosis and final treatment outcome of impacted maxillary canines. In this study, all the pretreatment and post-treatment data of the patients have gathered along with patient-related variables to identify links between these variables. The study inferred that Artificial intelligence could be used in dentistry to assist dental professionals. Some researchers made a model using the Artificial neural network to predict the necessity of extraction during an orthodontic treatment regime.

Data mining analysis done on the bulk of restorative data of patients revealed that differences in the material of restoration of tooth serve as important factors determining the lifespan of restoration. The strength of data mining lies in its ability to find causal relationships and comparisons that are innate in existing data.

A study done by Kakilehtoetal observed that the mean and median survival time (MST) of the amalgam restorations for the occlusal surface was 16.8 years within the 1960 cluster,
13.6 years within the 1970 cluster and 7.9 years within the 1980 cluster. For glass ionomer and composite resin restoration on the occlusal surface, MST was 4.9 years within the 1970 cluster and 7.3 years within the 1980 cluster. The observations were obtained by data mining analysis; the only role of the dental professionals was to collect and tabulate the data.

All the above studies proved the application of AI in the current dental field to diagnose and make prognosis through the exclusion of useful information from large amounts of medical records. So, Artificial intelligence is basically concentrated on making strong systems to facilitate dental professionals to make decisions as well as to help patients understand their diseases and their prognosis.

Recent advances in neural networks

Recently several variations of artificial neural networks have been reported, which include:

1. Convolutional Neural Networks (CNNs) for image classification challenges.
2. Dilated Convolutional Neural Networks (DCNNs) for semantic scene segmentation challenges.
3. Two main classes of CNN prevail for volumetric prediction in general.
4. Tiramisu.
5. Dilated convolutional neural networks (DCNNs) data.

• Tiramisu-based models such as U-net excel at predicting dose volumes that tend to be spatially consistent to anatomy, such as the dose volume to a prostate.
• Dilated Convolutional Neural Networks (DCNNs) utilize convolutions that skip over information during encoding to help extend their field of view. DCNNs can be useful for predicting doses that can be mobile to anatomy, as in head and neck cancer patients. Likely, these methods will also soon become standard in volumetric dose prediction for head and neck IMRT (Intensity-Modulated Radiation Therapy).

1.6.6 Fuzzy logic

Fuzzy logic is the science of thinking, reasoning, and inference that recognizes and uses the real-world phenomenon, and instead of assuming everything is black and white (conventional logic), fuzzy logic recognizes that in reality, most things would fall somewhere in between, that is varying shades of grey. Oral and dental diseases are common at every age, but patients ignore these problems. The reason is the fear of going to the dentist or the costly treatment. Ambara and colleagues designed a fuzzy logic-based expert system that is time, and cost-friendly, and consultation can be done without using tools that reduce fear of the patient. Hererra and coworkers used a fuzzy logic-based system that predicted the color change after tooth bleaching on the basis of the tooth's initial chrome values. The fuzzy logic system has rules corresponding to pre-bleaching shades of the well-known Vita commercial shade guide.

1.6.7 Evolutionary computation

Evolutionary computation is a general-purpose imaginary global optimization approach under the Neo-Darwinian paradigm. In the class of all the evolutionary algorithms, the Genetic Algorithm (GA) is extensively used. Holland first introduced it in 1975. A simple GA has three components: a population generator and selector, a fitness estimator, and three genetic operators (selection, mutation, and crossover). It has a series of successful applications in different disciplines like biology, medicine, and different branches of engineering. For example, its application in the medical field involves creating many random solutions to the problem at hand.

1.6.8 Hybrid intelligent systems

This combining system allows to fit in with common sense while using human-like reasoning mechanisms, extracting knowledge from raw data, dealing with uncertainty and imprecision, and learning to adapt to a rapidly changing and unknown environment. Moreover, the advantages of these technologies can be combined to produce hybrid intelligent systems which can work in a complementary manner. Many different hybrid systems are available, and the popular ones are ANNs for designing fuzzy systems, fuzzy systems for designing ANNs, and Genetic Algorithms for automatically training and generating neural network architecture.

1.6.9 Augmented reality and Virtual reality

It involves the superimposition of a computer-generated image on a user-made perspective of the natural world, accordingly giving a hybrid view. (26) Dentistry is a unique profession in the scope of medicine and is extremely demanding as requires the assimilation of large amounts of knowledge combined with the acquisition of clinical skills. (27)The invention of augmented reality has simplified the process of delivering aesthetic prostheses and meeting the patient's expectations. With the help of AI systems and augmented reality, the patient can try on a virtual prosthesis that can be altered till the patient is satisfied, and the final prosthesis is made exactly according to these specifications. (28)Virtual reality, on the other hand, is a computer-generated simulation of a three-dimensional image or environment that can be interacted with in a seemingly real or physical way by a person using special electronic equipment. AI systems, along with virtual reality, have been used not only to reduce dental anxiety but are also regarded as a powerful tool for non-pharmacological control of pain. (29)

Cosmetic dentistry is one such branch of dentistry where the treatment outcome can be virtually demonstrated to the patient. This not only motivates the patient but also guides the dentist to focus on the predetermined outcome. Virtual reality is a computer-generated simulation of a three-dimensional model that can be interacted with in a seemingly real environment. The AI systems, along with virtual reality, have been used not only as an educational tool but also as a method of distraction for non-pharmacological control of pain. (5)

A computer-generated re-enactment of a three-dimensional image or environment can be communicated within a natural or physical path by an individual utilizing unique electronic equipment. (29)AR is a more commonly used technology applied in various medical and dental science areas.

Some of the applications of AR in Dentistry include:

1. The oral and maxillofacial branch of dentistry is one of the complicated areas due to the complex anatomy of the craniofacial region. Any surgery in this area requires perfect planning with high precision, which is quite difficult. AR assists dental surgeons by providing clear graphical information of operative sites that is then modified from a data source.
2. The positioning of dental implants, which is one of the difficult steps in dental implantology, is made easy by graphically obtained results of AR. The AR system used in dental implantology is considered as most effective as it reduces the time and cost of the dental implant.
3. Used in orthognathic surgery by expansion in facial skeleton osteotomy via partial visual immersion employing a head-mounted display.
4. Besides all these applications, AR is also used in dental education by combining digital variables with real learning domains.
5. AR also made learning live anatomy easy by visualizing the operator's body using augmented mirrored images.

1.6.10 Genetic Algorithms

They have also gained success during the last decade as optimization methods for complex problems. They are stochastic search methods that are based on the principle of survival of the fittest in natural selection. It includes approaches such as mutation, inheritance, selection, and crossover to search for a better option for the problem. The greatest advantage of genetic algorithms over conventional methods is that it works on the basis of problem-solving instead of the analytical relations concept of conventional methods. Despite being a powerful optimization tool, it works on simple rules, which makes it easy to implement. Łodygowski T and coworkers used genetic algorithms for optimization of a dental implant system to reduce the problem of mechanical fracture and to provide long-term strength to the implant.

Another study done by Li H et al. used a genetic algorithm along with back propagation neural network to improve tooth color matching, which is one of the greatest challenges in prosthodontics dentistry. A recent study reported the genetic algorithm-based approach to detect dental caries in its early stages in order to avoid the severity of the decay. Also, a Genetic algorithm is employed in the reconstruction of missing parts of the tooth by optimizing a set of control points in computer-aided design. This study showed that there is a good scope of geometric modeling and optimization techniques using genetic algorithms to regulate the reconstructed surface and maintain the overall smoothness.

1.6.11 Receiver Operating Characteristic (ROC) curve

The area under the ROC curve (called AUC) is plotted as the true positive rate (TPR) on the y-axis and the false positive rate (FPR) on the x-axis. The higher the AUC, the better the algorithm is at classifying (e.g., disease vs. no disease); thus, an AUC=1 indicates perfect ability to distinguish between classes, an AUC=0.5 means no ability to distinguish between classes (complete overlap), and an AUC=0 indicates the worst result–all incorrect assignments.

1.6.12 Percent(%) accuracy

Percent accuracy is the proportion of correct predictions, determined by dividing the number of correct predictions (true positives + true negatives; TPs + TNs) by all observations (TPs+TNs + false positives and false negatives (FPs+FNs)). This metric is inadequate, however, when there is uneven class distribution (i.e., significant disparity between the sample sizes for each label).

1.6.13 Sensitivity and specificity

Sensitivity is synonymous with the TPR and "recall" (R) and measures the proportion of TPs measures the proportion of TNs that are correctly identified (TNs/(TNs+FPs)). Sensitivity that is correctly identified (TPs/(TPs+FNs)) Specificity is synonymous with TNR, and specificity is inversely proportional; as sensitivity increases, specificity decreases and vice versa.

1.6.14 Precision

(also called positive predictive value; PPV)
Precision is the proportion of positive identifications (e.g., presence of MDD) that are correctly classified by the algorithm (TPs/(TPs+FPs)). For example, precision=0.5 means that the algorithm correctly predicted MDD

50% of the time. An F1 score is a measure of an algorithm's accuracy that conveys the balance between precision and recall, calculated as 2*((precision*recall)/(precision+recall)). The best value of an F1 score is 1, and the worst is 0. F1 scores can be more useful than accuracy in studies with uneven class distributions.

1.7 Hierarchy

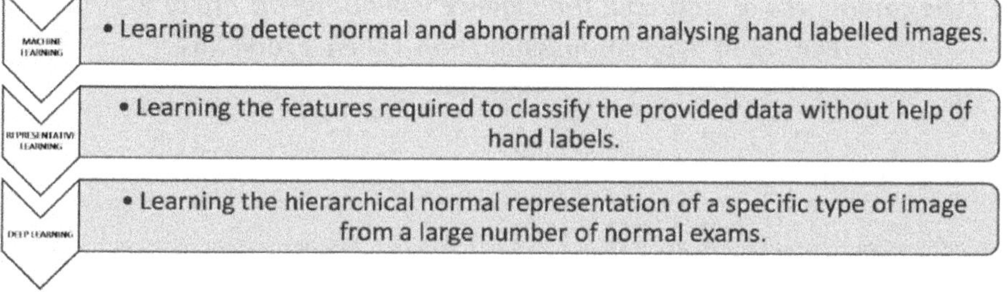

Figure 2 Hierarchy of AI

CHAPTER TWO

HISTORY AND EVALUATION

"The coming era of Artificial Intelligence will not be the era of war, but be the era of deep compassion, non-violence, and love."
-Amit Ray

2.1 Overview

To be informed about the history of artificial intelligence, it is necessary to go back to previous dates in Milat. (30) In the Ancient Greek era, it is proven that various ideas about humanoid robots have been carried out. An example is Daedelus, who is said to have ruled the mythology of the wind to try to create artificial humans. The emergence of artificial intelligence officially in history dates back to 1956. In 1956, at a conference on artificial intelligence session at Dartmouth College, AI was introduced for the first time. Marvin Minsky stated in his book "Stormed Search for Artificial Intelligence "that" the problem of artificial intelligence modeling within a generation will be solved. "

The first artificial intelligence applications were introduced during this period. These applications are based on logic theorems and chess games. The programs developed during this period were distinguished from the geometric forms used in intelligence tests, which led to the idea that intelligent computers could be created. Between 1965 and 1970, it could be called a dark period for artificial intelligence. The developments in artificial intelligence in this period are too few to be tested. The hasty and optimistic attitude due to the unrealistic expectations that have emerged has led to the idea that it will be easy to uncover the machines with intelligence. But this period was named a dark period on behalf of artificial intelligence because it did not succeed with the idea of creating intelligent machines by simply uploading data.

Between 1970 and 1975, artificial intelligence gained momentum. Thanks to the success achieved in artificial intelligence systems that have been developed and developed on subjects such as disease diagnosis, the basis of today's artificial intelligence have been established. During the period 1975-1980, they developed the idea that they could benefit from artificial intelligence through other branches of science such as psychology. Artificial Intelligence began to be used in large projects with practical applications in the 1980s. The next time the daylight is passed, artificial intelligence has been adapted to solve real-life problems. Even when users' needs are already met with traditional methods, the use of artificial intelligence has reached a much wider range thanks to more economical software and tools.

2.2 Milestones of AI with Chronological Order

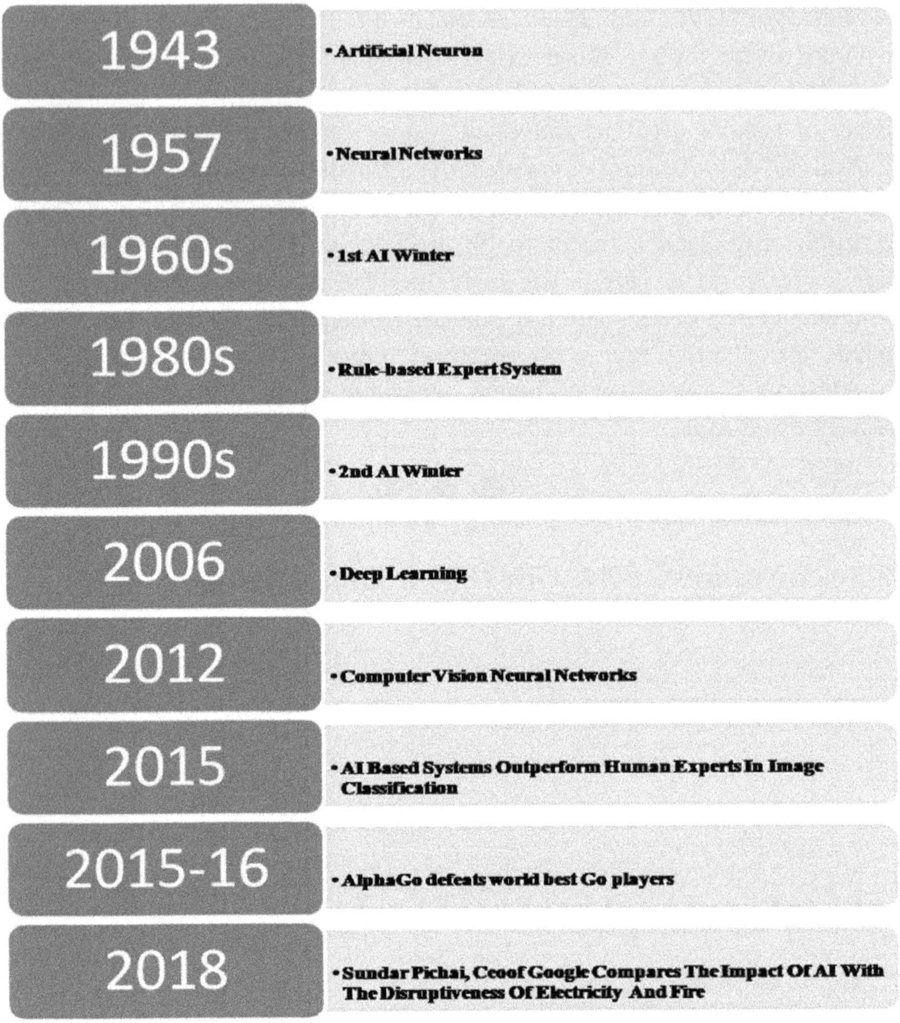

Year	Milestone
1943	• Artificial Neuron
1957	• Neural Networks
1960s	• 1st AI Winter
1980s	• Rule-based Expert System
1990s	• 2nd AI Winter
2006	• Deep Learning
2012	• Computer Vision Neural Networks
2015	• AI Based Systems Outperform Human Experts In Image Classification
2015-16	• AlphaGo defeats world best Go players
2018	• Sundar Pichai, Ceoof Google Compares The Impact Of AI With The Disruptiveness Of Electricity And Fire

Figure 3 Milestones of AI in chronological order

2.3 Timeline of History of AI

1206: Ebru İz Bin Rezzaz Al Jazeera, one of the pioneers of cybernetic science, has made water-operated automatic controlled machines.

1623: Wilhelm Schickard invented a mechanic and a calculator capable of four operations.

1672: Gottfried Leibniz developed a binary counting system that formed the abstract basis of today's computers.

1822-1859: Charles Babbage is a mechanical calculator. Ada Lovelace is regarded as the first computer programmer because of the work he has done with Babbage's punched cards on his machines. Lovelace's work includes algorithms.

1923: Karel Capek first introduced the robot concept in the theater play of Rossum's Universal Robots (RUR-Rossum's Universal Robots).

1931: Kurt Gödel introduced the deficiency theory, which is called by his own name.

1936: Konrad Zuse developed a programmable computer named Z1 named 64 K memory.

1946: ENIAC (Electronic Numerical Integrator and Computer), the first computer in a room size of 30 tons, started to work.

1948: Johnvon Neumann introduced the idea of self-replicating program.

1950: Alan Turing, founder of computer science, introduced the concept of the Turing Test.

1951: The first artificial intelligence programs for the Mark 1device were written.

1952: Machine learning

1956: The logic theorist (Logic Theory-LT) program for solving mathematical problems is introduced by Newell, Shaw, and Simon. The system is regarded as the first artificial intelligence system. The end of the 1950s - the beginning of the 1960s: A schematic network for machine translation was developed by Margaret Masterman et al.

1958: John McCarty of MIT created the LISP (list Processing language) language.

1960: JCR Licklider described the human-machine relationship in his work.

1962: Unimation was established as the first company to produce robots for the industrial field.

1965: An artificial intelligence program, ELIZA was written.

1966: The first animated robot "Shakey" was produced at Stanford University.

1971: A research resource on computers in Biomedicine was founded by Saul Amarel at Rutgers University.

1973: DARPA began the development of protocols called TCP /IP.

1974: The Internet began to be used for the first time.

1978: Herbert Simonearneda Nobel Prize for his limited Rationality Theory, which is an important work on Artificial Intelligence.

1981: IBM produced the first personal computer.

1993: Production of Cog, a human-looking robot at MIT, began.

1997: Deep Blue, named supercomputer defeated world-famous chess player Kasparov.

1998: Furby, the first artificial intelligence player, was driven to the market.

2000: Kismet, named robot which can use gestures and mimic movements in communication, is introduced.

2005: Asimo, the closest robot to artificial intelligence and human ability and skill, was introduced.

2010: Asimo is made to act using mind power.

CHAPTER THREE

GENERAL APPLICATIONS & APPLICATION IN HEALTH SCIENCES

"If we do it right, we might be able to evolve a form of work that taps into our uniquely human capabilities and restores our humanity. The ultimate paradox is that this technology may become a powerful catalyst that we need to reclaim our humanity."
-JohnHagel

3.1 In General

Weather Forecasting
Computer Vision
Game Playing
Recommendations
Robotics
NLP
Expert System
Handwritting Recognition
Image Recognition
Telecommunication
Aerospace
Medicine And Dentistry
AI Application Areas

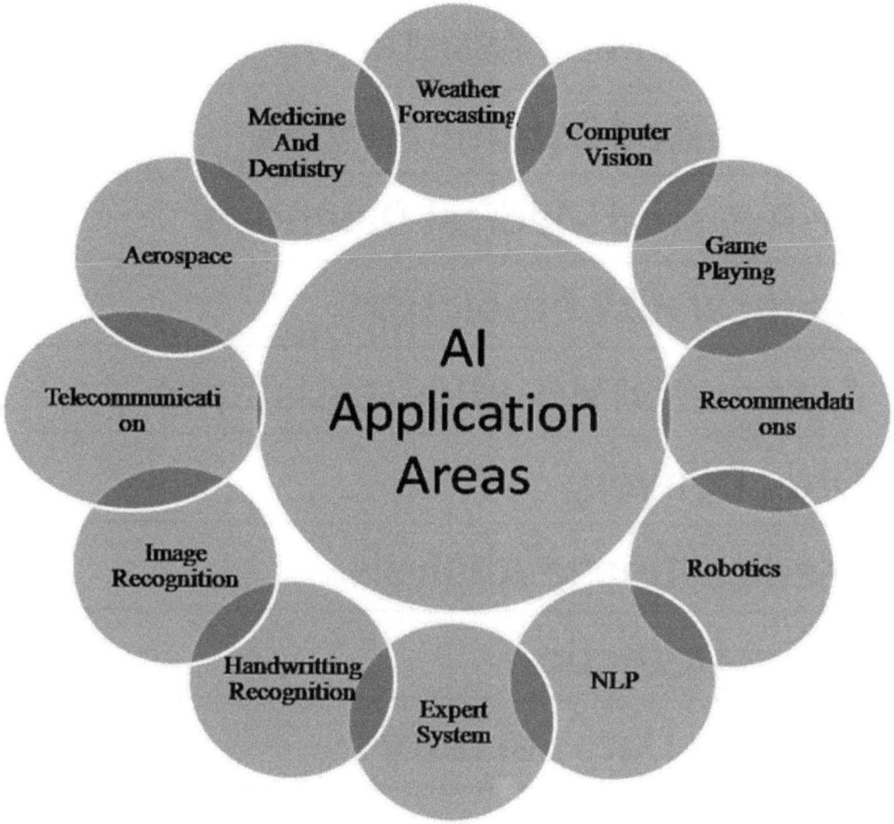

Figure 4 General applications of AI (31,32)

3.2 In Health Care

Virtual Nursing Assistants
AI- Assisted Robotic Surgery
AI- Assisted Medical Diagnosis
Medical Risk Prediction
Automated Workflow assistance
Drug Delivery
Medical Image Analysis
Fraud Detection
Medical Data Security
Clinical Trials

Figure 5 Application of AI in health care(33)

3.3 Dentistry In General

The important applications of AI in dentistry include:

1. In Dental Education:
With the recent incorporation of artificial intelligence in intelligent tutoring systems like the Unified Medical Language System (UMLS), there is a huge

improvement in the quality of feedback that the preclinical virtual patient provides the students.

2. ANN: It has sufficient precision for the design and chair-side manufacturing of dental prostheses based on digital image acquisition following tooth cusps assessment. It can have great potential in investigating the properties of dental materials such as chemical stability, wear resistance, and flexural strength.

3. Artificial Intelligence in Patient Management:
It can assist in coordinating regular appointments and alerts the patients and dentists about checkups whenever any genetic or lifestyle information indicates increased susceptibility to dental diseases (eg, periodontal screening for patients with diabetes and oral cancer screening for those who habitually use smoked or smokeless tobacco). It can also create a database about any relevant medical history or about any allergies that the patient may have. It can not only assist in clinical diagnosis and treatment but also provide emergency Tele assistance in cases of dental emergencies when the dental healthcare professional cannot be contacted.

4. Artificial intelligence in Radiology:
It can be integrated with imaging systems like MRI (magnetic resonance imaging) and CBCT (cone beam computed tomography) to identify minute deviations from normalcy that could have gone unnoticed by the human eye. This can also be used to accurately locate landmarks on radiographs, which can be used for cephalometric diagnosis. ML algorithm can detect a lymph node in the head and neck image as normal or abnormal provided it is trained Radiologistby analyzing thousands of such images which are labeled as normal or abnormal. (34)

ANN is found to act as a second opinion to locate the minor apical foramen, thereby enhancing the accuracy of working length determination by radiographs and in diagnosing proximal dental caries. It is also found to have sufficient sensitivity, specificity, and accuracy to be a model for vertical root fracture detection in digital radiography. (35)

Wang et al. first presented an article that used DCNNs in the diagnosis and analysis of dental radiographs. In addition, Miki et al. conducted research that focused on classifying tooth types in dental cone-beam CT images via an automated method of DCNN. (36)

Recently, Lee et al. studied DCNN using a computer-assisted diagnosis (CAD) system for the detection of osteoporosis on panoramic radiographs. The DCNN CAD system was compared to the experienced oral and maxillofacial radiologist, and the results showed high agreement between the two.

5. Dar-Odehetal conducted a study to utilize ANN to predict rather unclear entities of diseases termed recurrent aphthous stomatitis. (37)

6. Artificial Intelligence in Prosthetic Dentistry:

In order to provide an ideal esthetic prosthesis for the patient various factors like anthropological calculations, facial measurements, ethnicity, and patient preferences have been integrated by a design assistant, RaPid, for use in prosthodontics. Rapidly integrates computer-aided design, knowledge-based systems, and databases, employing a logic-based representation as a unifying medium. With the help of Artificial Intelligence, the computer can actually guide the dentist during the entire procedure of making a digital impression and aid in making an ideal impression.

7. Artificial Intelligence in Orthodontics:

Diagnosis and treatment planning can be done by the analysis of radiographs and photographs by intraoral scanners and cameras. This eliminates the necessity for making a patient impression, as well as several laboratory steps, and the results are usually much more accurate compared to human perception. The tooth movement and final treatment outcome can be predicted by using algorithms and statistical analysis. (14) It can also be used to provide orthodontic consultations to general practitioners for the alignment of crowded lower teeth. (38)

Seok-Ki Junga and Tae-Woo Kimb conducted a study to construct an artificial intelligence expert system for the diagnosis of extractions using neural network machine learning and to evaluate the performance of this mode. This study suggested that artificial intelligence expert systems with neural network machine learning could be useful in orthodontics. (36)

8. Pain assessment:

Xiao-SuHuetal conducted a study where an artificial neural network (3-layer) achieved an optimal classification accuracy of 80.37% for pain and no pain discrimination. (39)

9. Head and neck cancer:

Ibragimov and Xing were the first to attempt the use of CNNs for the segmentation of organs at risk from head and neck cancer CT images. Their results confirmed that CNNs well-generalize the intensity appearance of objects with recognizable boundaries, whereas additional information may be required for CNN-based segmentation for the objects with poorly recognizable boundaries. (40) Another study was conducted which showed that genetic programming (GP) performed the best in oral cancer prognosis when the features selected are smoking, drinking, chewing, histological differentiation of SCC, and co-gene p63. It was also found that the GP outperformed the SVM and LR in oral cancer prognosis. GP is also proven to be applicable in drug discovery. (41) Fuzzy sets have been used to predict cervical lymph node metastasis in carcinoma of the tongue, for the prognosis of nasopharyngeal carcinoma, outcome prediction in esophageal cancer, and for the prediction of oral cancer susceptibility. (42) The neural network may be of value for the identification of individuals with a high risk of oral cancer or precancer for further clinical examination or health education. (38)

10. In periodontics

Lee et al. developed an architecture based on DCNN that consists of 16 convolution layers and two fully connected layers. The accuracy of their architecture in detecting periodontitis of premolars and molars was 81.0% and 76.7%, respectively.

Further, Rana et al. presented an autoencoder framework with convolutional layers to segment gingival diseases from oral images. This model successfully distinguishes between inflamed and healthy gingiva. (36) ANN can also effectively be used in classifying patients into aggressive periodontitis and chronic periodontitis group based on their immune response profile. Therefore ANNs can be employed for accurate diagnosis of AgPorCP by using relatively simple and conveniently obtained parameters, like leukocyte counts in peripheral blood. (43)

11. Patcus. R et al. conducted a study to evaluate the facial attractiveness of treated cleft patients and controls by artificial intelligence (AI) and to compare these results with panel ratings performed by lay people, orthodontists, and oral surgeons and found that the results were

comparable with the average scores of cleft patients seen in all three rating groups (with an especially strong agreement to both professional panels) but overall lower for control cases. (44)

12. Patcus. R et al. conducted another observational study which illustrates that artificial intelligence (convolutional neural networks) might be considered to score facial attractiveness and apparent age in orthognathic patients. (45)

13. Forensic dental imaging:
Personal Identification System Using Dental Panoramic Radiograph based on Meta_Heuristic Algorithm was reported to have an identification percentage approaching 97.7%. (46)

14. GAs and ANN are promising tools for predicting the sizes of unerupted canines and premolars with greater accuracy in the mixed dentition period and can also be optimized for predicting tooth surface loss which is a universal problem that involves an irreversible, multifactorial, non-carious, physiologic, pathologic, or functional loss of dental hard tissues. (38)

15. Another study was conducted with the objective of developing a decision support system for predicting the degree of color change after in-office tooth whitening by using colorimetric values. The patients' post-treatment color was largely close to the system prediction. (47)

	PUBLICATION YEAR	STUDY	DETAIL	ARTIFICIAL INTELLIGENCE TECHNOLOGY USED
RADIOLOGY	2018	Lee et al.	Diagnosis of caries	Deep Learning network
ORTHODONTICS	2016	Jung and Kim	Diagnosis of Orthodontic extraction	Artificial neural network
	2018	Thanathornwong	All clinical decision support	Bayesian networks
	2018	Patcas et al.	Treatment outcome analysis	Convolutional neural network
PERIODONTICS	2018	Lee et al.	Diagnosis and Predictionof periodontally compromised teeth	Convolutional neural network
	2018	Feres et al.	Differentiation between aggressive And chronic periodontitis	Support vector machine
ORAL MEDICINE	1995	Speight et al.	Risk prediction of Oral Cancer	Artificial neural network
	2018	Kim et al.	Prediction of MRONJ	Artificial neural network, Support vector machine, Logistic regression, and decision tree

Table 1 Summary of application of AI in dentistry

3.4. In SARS-CoV-2

3.4.1 In SARS-CoV-2 Screening:

Near the beginning, diagnosis of any disease, whether contagious or non-infectious, is a critical obstacle for premature care to save more lives. The rapid diagnostic and screening approach seeks to prevent and speed up the eventual diagnosis of increased diseases such as COVID-19. By being more cost-effective compared to the traditional approach, the creation of a specialist assists in the current organization of SARS-CoV-2 carrier identification screening and management. Machine learning and artificial intelligence are enhanced by the diagnostic and program procedure of the recognized patient using radio imaging technology similar to X-ray, computed tomography, and blood sample data.

The researcher and expert should use scientific images such as CT scans and X-rays as normal methods to boost conventional screening and diagnosis. Sadly, after the high eruption of the SARS-CoV-2 pandemic, the efficiency of such tools is moderate. In this observation, studies (Ardakanietal.2020) show the capacity of artificial intelligence and machine learning instruments by proposing a novel approach with a fast and true COVID-19 diagnostic mechanism using deep learning. The research reveals the analysis of 108 COVID-19 contaminated patients on 1020 CT images using an expert approach using AI and ML, along with viral pneumonia of 86 patients, that convolution neural network as a tool for radiologists results in 87.11%, 82.21% of precision accuracy, in that order.

With the new approach, automatic identification of COVID-19 based on an AI algorithm (Ozturk et al. 2020), current researchers have created a tool to improve the precision of the diagnosis of COVID-19. With the help of X-ray images, 129 infected patients with 498 without findings and 498 records of cases of pneumonia are included in the built model.

Many clusters proved the applicability of the proficient model to quickly and accurately verify the screening process to help radiology. Researchers have identified 11 main related indices (total protein, bilirubin, basophil, creatine kinase isoenzyme, platelet distribution distance, GLU, calcium, creatinine, lactate dehydrogenase, potassium, and magnesium) after examining 253 Wuhan clinical blood samples, which may help COVID-19 as an important screening discrimination tool for healthcare professionals (Sun et al.2020; Wuet al.2020).

Overall, the study provides confirmation of the expert system's implementation; the primary goal was to design rapid diagnosis along with the increasing results. In this concept, the detection reduces the progression of the condition and saves some time for the specialist to adapt the next observation and save lives which decreases the cost of medicine. Nevertheless, a machine learning classification algorithm was used on relevant data for most of the analyzed papers.

3.4.2 SARS-Cov-2Tracing

Anticipation of the extent of the illness by contact monitoring is the next crucial phase after an individual is analyzed and confirmed with COVID-19. According to the WHO, the virus spreads primarily by contact transfer from one person to another through sweat and running nose (WHO2020a). Touch monitoring is an important healthcare method people use to disrupt the transmission of the disease chain to control the spread of COVID-19 (WHO2020b). The person tracing tool is used to classify and handle public newly showing to attaint COVID-19 infected people to prevent additional dissemination.

Usually, the treatment identifies the infected organism with a 14-days go after the following exposure. This method would break the COVID-19 chain of the novel coronavirus and reduce the spate by presenting a greater potential for successful helping and controls to minimize the severity of the recent deadly disease. In order to create a digital communication monitoring mechanism with the smartphone application, many infected countries use various technologies such as Global Positioning System (GPS) network-based API, Bluetooth, contact information, social graph, and mobile tracking data. The automated tracing procedure can be real-time and easier.

These automated technologies are intended to capture data from individual apps that will be processed by artificial intelligence software to track an individual. A study has demonstrated the use of artificial intelligence propelling the pace of contact tracing against COVID-19 diseases.

After applying the graph theory to data on epidemics of infectious animal diseases, mainly shipping records between each farm, the consequential pictorial properties produced by the planned model can be used to allow contact tracing to be used effectively to improve contact tracing.

Though, presently there are restrictions when resolving situations, anonymity, data management, and still data safety breaches. Many nations, such as Israel, have “passed the emergency law on mobile phone records” to fight this disease. In the middle of the worldwide touch tracing applications, some countries' apps have broken the confidentiality act and have been reported as risky before they do the job properly by supplementing the manual tracing process.

3.4.3 Forecasting Of Disease

A new model, which forecasts and predicts 1 to 7 days to the front of the generally infected COVID-19 individuals in Brazilian states, has been suggested to use the stacking ensemble with the assist vector regression algorithm on the growing infected COVID-19 cases of this country's results, thereby extending the short-term prediction loop to advise the professionals to compensate for the disease (Ribeiro etal.2020).

Using a machine learning classifier named XGBoost on mammographic factor datasets, recent studies have indicated a new method. After applying the algorithm, the experts found that some of the distinctiveness of the 74 experimental and blood test samples (lactic dehydrogenase (LDH), lymphocyte, high-sensitivity C-reactive protein) in estimating and calculating the total number of COVID-19 patients with extreme mortality rates has a median accuracy of 91% (Yanetal.2020).

On the other hand, in identifying the majority of patients in need of intensive medical treatment, the comparatively greater importance of single lactic dehydrogenase tends to be a crucial factor, such that the degree of LDH involved in various lung illnesses, such as asthma, bronchitis, and pneumonia.

The proposed method used the assessment rule to allow patients to be manageable for intensive care and to potentially reduce the rate of transience in order to easily estimate and forecast infectious people at the greatest risk. Using a deep learning algorithm for the long term, a Canadian-based forecasting model was developed using time series.

A key factor in predicting the short-term memory network trajectory was established in the studies, with an end-point prediction of the latest SARS-CoV-2 outbreak in Canada and around the world (Chimmulaand Zhang2020). For this SARS-CoV-2 outbreak in Canada, the proposed end-point model estimate will be around June 2020 (JHU 2020); the prediction was likely to be accurate as newly infected cases dropped rapidly and proved the applicability of the expert approach to predicting and forecasting the next pandemic/epidemic by re-establishing key aspects of veiling.

In order to combine the accuracy of the wavelet-based forecasting model with the optimized autoregressive moving average time series model (Chakraborty and Ghosh 2020), the real-time forecasting model was proposed. The model solves the problem by designing short-term SARS-CoV-2 forecasts for various countries as a temporary warning module for each target country to assist healthcare professionals and policymakers.

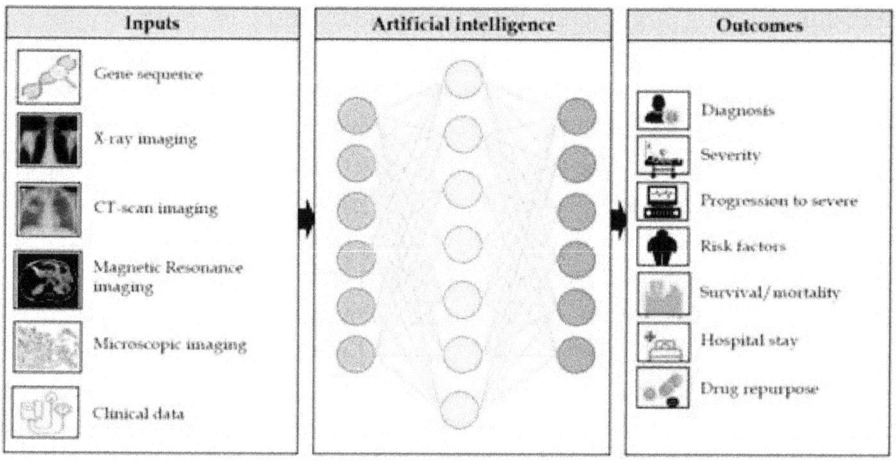

Figure6 Application of AI to fighting COVID-19

3.4.4 In SARS-CoV-2 Medicines and Vaccines

After the beginning of the coronavirus epidemic, scientists and healthcare professionals around the world have been encouraged to develop a potential solution to the development of drugs and vaccines for the SARS-CoV-2 pandemic, and ML/AI technology is an enthralling path. With regard to the likelihood of drug selection for the treatment of infected patients, it is important to provide an urgent review of the existing old, marketable medicines for new SARS-CoV-2 carriers in human beings.

Taiwanese researchers are designing a new strategy for increasing the production of a new drug (Ke et al., 2020). The study revealed eight drugs,i.e., gemcitabine, vismodegib, and clofazimine, using the deep neural network on eighty-year-old drugs with COVID-19 therapeutic potential after two datasets were added to the ML and AI technology-based model (one using 3C-like protease restriction and other data keeping cases of infection with SARS-CoV, SARS-Cov-2, influenza, and human immune-deficiency virus). Additionally, five other drugs, such as salinomycin, homoharringtonine, chloroquine, tilorone, and boceprevir, have also been shown to be operational in the AI laboratory setting.

Researchers from the USA and Korea jointly suggested a novel molecule transformer-drug target interaction model address the need for an antiviral drug to cure the COVID-19 virus. The report contrasts AutoDock Vina, a free collaborative screening and molecular docking programmer, to the suggested model, using a deep learning algorithm on COVID-19 3C-like proteins approved by the FDA, with 3410 new drugs available on the market. The findings found that the best treatment for COVID-19, followed by remdesivir, was a common antiretroviral medication used to treat HIV called atazanavir (Kdof94.94 nM)(Kdof113.13nM).

In addition, the findings showed that some drugs for viral proteinase therapy, such as darunavir, ritonavir, and lopinavir, were illuminated. It was also observed that for the medication of COVID-19 human patients, many antiviral compounds such as Kaletra may be used. An antiviral drug was developed by a group of researchers from the USA to cure the Ebola virus. The study was first made in 2014 (Ekins et al. 2014), beginning with the ML and AI pharmacophore-based statistical study of the small size of in vitro infected carriers of Ebola viruses. The study suggested a widely used amodiaquine and chloroquine complex for the treatment of the malaria virus. In addition, a blend of numerical screening methods with docking applications and machine learning was introduced after finding a decade of drug development focused on ML and AI technologies to pick supplementary medicine to investigate SARS-CoV-2 (Ekins et al.2020). Researchers are looking at the successful management of Ebola (Ekins et al. 2020) and the experience of the Zika virus (Ekins et al. 2016), and the same model can also be used to classify COVID-19 drugs and a potential pandemic of the virus. It was noted that in combination with the docking application, the use of machine software was more effective in forecasting the reusability of an existing old COVID-19 medication and greatly decreasing the amount of a risk factor in creating a more cost-effective drug operation. During this emergency, the use of ML and AI will improve the drug production process by reducing the time slot for the courier to explore an alternative therapy and remedy by depending on a high chance of the efficacy, manageability, and clinical knowledge of the current medicine compound.The finite resources of stable hybrid data and real-life deployment of the programs were the concerns and problems found in this area.

3.4.5 Methods Used in Predicting COVID-19

Recurrent Neural Networks (RNN)

Deep learning speculates that a deep sequential or hierarchical model is more effective than shallow models (Bengio 2009) in classification or regression functions. There are implied states distributed over time in recurrent neural networks, and this helps them to retain a lot of previous knowledge. Due to their ability to handle variable length sequential data, they are most widely used in forecasting applications (Graves2013).

There is a major drawback to recurrent COVID-19 confirmed, active, recovered, and tested cases in India 108 6 Visualization and Prediction of COVID-19 Using AI and ML neural networks that they do not respond to the gradient disappearance or gradient explosion problem and can only store short-term memory and have only hidden layer activation functions in the previous step (Hochreiter and Schmidhuber 1997).

Long Short-Term Memory (LSTM) and Its Variants

It is known that LSTMs are among the most efficient solutions for prediction operations, and based on the different highlighted features present in the dataset, they forecast future predictions. With LSTMs, knowledge travels through elements known as cell states. LSTMs may recall or miss details correctly. The data obtained over progressive stretches of time is known to be the data from time series, and LSTMs are typically used as a rigorous means of calculating these data values.

The model converts the previous veiled state to the appropriate stage of the arrangement in this style of architecture. Long short-term memory cells (Hochreiter and Schmidhuber 1997) are used for long-term memory retrieval RNNs, while RNNs can retain only a small amount of information. The problems of the gradient disappearing and the bursting gradient (Bengio et al. 1994) plaguing RNN are resolved by LSTMs. LSTM cells are similar to RNN, with memory blocks replaceable by hidden modules.

Deep LSTM / Stacked LSTM

The regular LSTM extension we have defined above is stacked LSTM (Graves et al. 2013), also known as Deep LSTM. There are several hidden layers and several memory cells on the stacked LSTM. The depth of the neural network is improved by the stacking of multiple layers, where each layer has some information and transfers it to the next. The top LSTM layer supplies the previous layer with sequence information and so on. For each time step, it produces a different output instead of a single output for all time steps.

Bidirectional LSTM (Bi-LSTM)

Inputs are processed by traditional RNNs in only one direction and ignore the possible knowledge that they provide. By following the bidirectional topology of LSTM (Schusterand Paliwal 1997), this issue is solved. By keeping both past and future information into account, bidirectional LSTM (Bi-LSTM) excludes absolute temporal time information. Periodic secret RNN neurons are separated into forwarding and backward states in which forward state neurons are not bound to backward states and vice versa. The design without the backward states is identical to the normal unidirectional RNN. There is no need to provide extra time delays as used for this process in standard RNN.

CHAPTER FOUR

APPLICATIONS IN ORAL MEDICINE AND ORAL RADIOLOGY

"By far, the greatest danger of Artificial Intelligence is that people conclude too early that they understand it."
-Eliezer Yudkowsky

4.1 Oral Medicine In General

Correct diagnosis is the key to a successful clinical practice. In this regard, adequately trained neural networks can be a boon to diagnosticians, especially in conditions having multi-factorial etiology. (38)Virtual dental assistants, which are based on AI, can perform various functions and tasks with greater accuracy in the dental clinic, with minimal errors and less workforce compared to humans. In departments such as oral medicine and radiology, oral pathology can be used to arrange appointments, manage insurance and article works, and help diagnose or treatment. It is very helpful in notifying the dentist regarding patients' complete medical and dental history as well as other oral hygiene habits, food and diet habits, and habits such as alcoholism and smoking. In dental emergencies, the patient has an option of emergency Tele assistance, especially when the practitioner is unavailable. Thus, comprehensive virtual data of the patients can be generated, which will help in providing ideal treatment for the patient in long run. (48) The diagnoses and treatment of lesions of the oral cavity can be screened and classified into suspicious altered mucosa undergoing premalignant and malignant changes with the help of AI. The genetic predisposition of oral cancer for a large population might be accurately predicted using AI. Images of the oral cavity for remote interpretation by specialists can be captured using Mobile Mouth Screening Anywhere (MeMoSA) app.

4.2 Oral Radiology In General

Background

Image recognition using AI systems has shifted from a science tale into reality within the radiology practice in the last 20 years. Practicing radiologists need to understand both the value and the pitfalls, weaknesses, and potential errors that may occur when an AI product performs image analysis. (48) Radiologists should be familiar with AI terminology and hierarchy. Radiology programs should begin to integrate health informatics, computer science, and statistics courses into their curriculum. To train the radiologist for logic, statistics, and data science and be aware of other sources of information such as genomics and biometrics, in so far as they can integrate data from disparate sources with a patient's clinical condition. Radiologists should understand the challenges related to the preparation of training datasets for supervised learning.

While these algorithms are powerful, they are often brittle and may give inappropriate answers when presented with images outside of their knowledge set. (49) This includes images with technical artifacts such as movement or beam hardening or images obtained with inappropriate techniques. For example, an algorithm evaluating brain CTs may work perfectly for long stretches, but then a new software upgrade to the CT occurs, or a new CT machine comes online, and all of a sudden, the algorithm produces faulty results. To alleviate this concern, in many modalities, new protocols for standardized imaging should be adopted with AI in mind, similar to guidelines proposed for image acquisition to enable quantitative analysis. (50) AI is used for more than image analysis. It is a powerful tool to identify patterns, predict behavior or events, or categorize objects. In the near future, these none image analysis tools may dramatically affect radiology. For example, these tools have the potential to improve radiology departmental workflow through precision scheduling, identification of patients most at risk of missing appointments, and empowering individually tailored exam protocols. Perhaps most anxiety-provoking for radiologists, AI may enable programs that use radiologists and their work as data, identifying details of each radiologist's practice pattern and even categorizing them, enabling the creation of a sophisticated radiology report card.

AI gives added advantage in head and neck imaging due to its distinctive ability to learn and maybe assimilate with other imaging modalities like CBCT and MRI to work out minute deviations from normality that would have gone unrecognized by the human eye.

Illustrations including the definite location of landmarks on radiographs aid in the detection of vertical root fractures, cephalometric analysis, diagnosis of maxillary sinusitis on panoramic radiographs, and Waters' radiographs to detect Sjogren syndrome on CT. Economically these might be translated into far better patient care. The incorporation of Artificial Intelligence in 3D printing helps to manufacture in its prefabrication stage. Predicting the possible failure of the printing process and resolving the overhang problem can be achieved using AI software [33]. With Intelligent algorithms, solutions to any problem can be found quickly enough, thereby enabling 3D printers to perform effectively and guiding to resolve of any quality issues. Some future recommendations for radiologists will be they should be familiar with AI terminology and hierarchy, should begin to integrate health informatics, computer science, and statistics courses in their curriculum, train the radiologist in logic, statistics, data science, and be aware of other sources of information such as genomics and biometrics, to integrate data from disparate sources with a patient's clinical condition. Radiologists should understand the challenges related to the preparation of training data sets for supervised learning.

In head-and-neck imaging modalities, AI provides additional leverage owing to its unique ability to learn. It can be integrated with imaging systems such as magnetic resonance imaging and cone-beam computed tomography to identify minute deviations from normalcy that could have gone unnoticed by the human eye. Examples include the accurate location of landmarks on radiographs, which can assist a cephalometric diagnosis. ANN is found to act as a second opinion to locate the minor apical foramen, thereby enhancing the accuracy of working length determination by radiographs and in diagnosing proximal dental caries. It is also found to have sufficient sensitivity, specificity, and accuracy to be a model for vertical root fracture detection in digital radiography.

Scenarios and the classes of use cases of AI in radiology

Clinical workflow	Types of applications	Classes of use cases
Triage scenario	Detection	For workflow optimization and quality assurance
Replacement scenario	Segmentation	Separate normal from not normal
Add on scenario	classification	Grading and classification of images Computer aided detection Radiomics Computer assisted reporting

Table 2 Scenarios and the classes of use cases of AI in radiology

Different scenarios:

Different scenarios used in the clinical workflow are triage (34), replacement, and add-on, which are based on the conceptual framework developed by Bossuyt et al.(51) Triage scenario adapted form is used as a screening tool to sort examinations based on the probability of disease being positive or negative according to AI. For example, AI will assess the not interpreted x-rays for the highest probability of disease determined by an algorithm according to the content of images or other data available and determine which examination should be interpreted first.

In a replacement scenario, AI may replace radiologists if results are consistently more accurate, rapid, reproducible, and easier to obtain. The most common application of it is an estimation of bone age by AI software. AI is found to consistently provide better performance than a radiologist in bone age estimation. An Add-on scenario may use AI in a subgroup of patients where the existing clinical pathway is dependent on the radiologist's interpretation. This tool is applied only if the imaging findings warrant a time-consuming application best left to ML algorithms.

? **Types of application**

This can be divided into

1. Detection: To identify an anomaly within an image (eg, a nodule);
2. Segmentation: To isolate a structure from the remainder of the study (eg, defining the boundary of an organ); and
3. Classification: To assign an image or lesion within an image representing a category (eg, is the presence or absence of pulmonary embolism on a CT scan).

? **Classes of use Cases**

1. To Separate normal from abnormal
2. For workflow optimization and quality assurance: AI can detect minor changes in the images saving the observers time, and also can help by retrieving previous data of the patient or finding similar findings in other images providing a list of possibilities.
3. Grading and classification of images: The ACR Reporting and Data Systems (RADS) provide assessment structure and classification for reporting inpatient imaging. (52)
4. Radiomics process extracts a large number of quantitative features from medical images. Though it can potentially be applied to any medical condition, it is currently applied mostly in the quantification of tumor phenotype and the development of decision support tools in oncology. (53)

Natural language processing (NLP): NLP is commonly defined as the conversion of unstructured text into a structured form to allow for the automated extraction of information, synonymous with text mining or information extraction. AI analyses a large amount of unstructured information in full-text radiology reports extracting the potentially invaluable source of information for clinical care quality improvement and research, which would have been a challenge otherwise due to the varied and individual reporting styles of narrative reports. (54)

? **Outputs of artificial intelligence in radiology**

Preprocessing

Image operations such as image enhancement, image normalization, and noise removal are often performed in a preprocessing step. (55) Image enhancement is a process where the image is adjusted so that the image is more suitable for either visualization or further analysis. Specific examples include removal of noise from the image, sharpening of the image, image intensity adjustments, or facilitating easier object detection (image segmentation). A variety of methods exist for obtaining such goals. Filtering with morphological operators may be used as a method for removing small objects in the image and correcting non-uniform background illumination.

Filtering may be performed using a structuring element of a customizable size and shape. A larger structuring element will remove larger objects than a smaller structuring element. In the case of correcting nonuniform background illumination, all objects in the image are removed, and the background intensity can subsequently be assessed and subtracted from the original image. Median filtering may be used for, for example, noise removal in images. The median filtering approach works by assigning the output pixel value to the median value of the neighboring input pixels. This approach removes outliers in the pixel values, as they would be far from the median value neighboring pixel values. Histogram equalization, also known as image normalization, may be used for performing contrast adjustments to the image so that the intensity values of the image span the entire intensity range. Furthermore, this larger span of intensity values allows for sharper differences between dark and bright regions.

In the field of image acquisition, it is also possible to encounter periodic noise in the images, which typically originate from electrical and/or electromechanical interference that affect the image acquisition. To remove the periodic noise, it is necessary to determine its parameters. These are typically assessed by analyzing the Fourier spectrum of the image. This periodic noise produces frequency spikes that can be easily detected, and when sufficiently pronounced, automated analysis can be invoked to ease the burden of determining the input parameters.

Segmentation

Image segmentation is an important step in many areas of the medical imaging field. This can be characterized as a process where objects or regions of interest are subdivided within the image. The subdivision or segmentation should hence be stopped when the region of interest or object has been isolated.

Segmentation of images is one of the most demanding tasks, and its accuracy is fundamental for subsequent analysis failures or successes. Segmentation algorithms are often based on either image intensity value similarities or image intensity value discontinuities. In the first case, segmentation is based on subdividing images into objects or regions of interest which appear to have similar intensity values based on a set of predefined criteria. In the second case, the segmentation is based on subdividing the image by following abrupt changes in the intensities. Within the segmentation of images using intensity discontinuities, there exist three basic types of approaches: point, line, and edge detection.

With respect to point and line detection, these techniques involve the detection of isolated points or straight lines in a given image, respectively, and are, of course, of importance in image segmentation in general. However, edge detection is by enlarging the most utilized method for detecting intensity value discontinuities. This is because an edge, in this case, can be described as an arbitrarily curved line, and especially in medical imaging, it is often so that we are not interested in detecting either points or straight lines. For edge detection, first derivatives are used as they have properties that necessitate that they are zero in regions of the image with constant intensity and non-zero and numerically correlated to the degree of intensity change in regions with variable intensities.

For the segmentation of images using intensity value similarities, thresholding is often used. Basic thresholding enjoys widespread use due to its simplicity of implementation and intuitive properties. In the most basic setting, a threshold value can be determined by trial and error and subsequently end up with a value that fits the purpose as judged by the user. Alternatively, a threshold value can be assessed by the visual inspection of a histogram of the image. These two proposed methods are, of course, highly user-dependent, so it is often advisable to utilize an algorithm that automatically chooses a threshold value based on the image data in question.

Object detection

Object detection using bounding boxes is often used in conjunction with deep learning neural network algorithms and has been implemented in medical images to detect an atomical structure in computed tomography (CT) scans. This technique is utilized for identifying one or multiple regions of interesting images. It could be utilized for the automated detection of gallstones in patients while also locating the position of the liver and spine in the image.

Applications in maxillofacial radiology (SUMMARY)

As the easiest fields for the evaluation of the efficiency of the application of AI are diagnostics of lung nodules and breast cancer screening, most of the research involving radiology is focused on it. The following aspect of dental-maxillofacial radiology has been researched with respect to AI:

1. Interpretation of radiographic lesions and automated interpretation of dental radiographs.
2. Using the radiologists' work as data, AI may enable programs to identify details of individual radiologists' practice patterns and categorize them to create a sophisticated radiology report card.
3. Caries detection: Logicon Caries Detector™ program (Logicon Inc., USA) is designed to assist dentists in the detection and characterization of proximal caries (56)
4. Diagnosis of vertical root fractures on CBCT images of endodontically treated and intact teeth
5. To stage tooth development
6. Computer-based digital subtraction imaging
7. Computer-assisted image analysis is useful to visualize and evaluate the bone architecture directly from the dental panoramic radiograph (57)
8. 3-dimensional orthodontics visualization using patient model sand OPGs
9. Bone density evaluation to predict osteoporosis using OPGS (58)
10. Automatic segmentation of mandibular canal (59)

Gerlach reported accuracy of automatic segmentation of the mandibular canal by the AAM and ASM methods is inadequate for use in clinical practice.

11. Forensic dental imaging: Personal Identification System Using Dental Panoramic Radiograph based on Meta_Heuristic Algorithm reported to have 97.7% precision
12. Dental biometrics

The Butterfly iQ

The Butterfly iQ is an innovative pocket-sized ultrasound device developed by the Butterfly Network. It utilizes capacitive micro-machined ultrasound transducer (CMUT)/ complementary metal oxide semiconductor-based parts in the ultrasonic probe. It differentiates itself from all other competitors by utilizing silicon chip CMUTs instead of using conventional piezoelectric crystal-based transducers. The CMUT has a much wider bandwidth compared to the piezoelectric transducers that are tuned to oscillate at specific frequencies.

A CMUT can thus be used to detect and emit many different frequencies, and as a result, a CMUT can be utilized for whole-body imaging. A major future area of application for the Butterfly iQ is interfacing with AI. The company has announced that this is a direction it will investigate by feeding the uploaded images from the users to a deep learning algorithm. The AI's aim is to enable the software to provide guidance to the user both during image interpretation and during image acquisition. Such AI capabilities could dramatically expand the application of the device into different realms of use. In one setting, the company envisions that in low-resource settings, AI-guided interpretations and guidance will be valuable. In another setting, the low cost of the device combined with possible AI-guided capabilities may entail that it can be offered as a personal medical device. The deep learning algorithms of the Butterfly network are used to power their computer vision applications. By training these on enough images related to a medical condition, their program learns how to scan the correct regions of the patient's body and can distinguish normal from abnormal tissue. Currently, most of the image processing and analysis is taking place in the cloud and not on the device or local networks. The ease of using devices like Butterfly iQ and the low cost of obtaining each image makes it attractive and fast to collect a large number of images for analysis. It is envisioned that this device would be available at retailers, including pharmacies or clinics, and the images captured with the device can be sent to a doctor for further analysis, similar to telehealth applications. The connected and automated nature of the device would also enable a diagnosis to be delivered almost instantaneously instead of weeks of delay and waiting.

4.3 Bone Diseases

In recent years, medical technology and effective interventions have led to an aging population. This means that while we live longer, we are increasingly prone to new types of conditions. Skeletal conditions and low bone mineral density (BMD) are high on this list and have been projected to grow and potentially add to mortality rates.

STUDY ON DIAGNOSIS OSTEOPOROSIS	TECHNIQUE	KEYFEATURES
Tassoker et al [60]	Deep Learning(DL)	• Female patients over 50 years of age were labeled as C1, C2, and C3 depending on mandibular cortical index(MCI) as shown in figure 7
		• According to this index; C1:presence of a smooth and sharp mandibular cortex(normal); C2: resorption cavities at endosteal margin and 1to3-layer stratification (osteopenia); C3:completely porotic cortex(osteoporosis). • The dataset C1-C2-C3 has an accuracy rate of 81.14% with AlexNET; the dataset C1-C2 hasan accuracy rate of 88.94% with GoogleNET;the datasetC1-C3 has an accuracy rate of 98.56% with AlexNET; and the dataset C1-(C2+C3) has an accuracy rate of 92.79% with GoogleNET indicating highest accuracy was obtained in differentiationof C3 and C1.
Kavithaet al[61]	Histogram based automatic clustering (HAC) algorithm with a Support vector machine (SVM)	• HAC-SVM method in combination with CAD system to measure Mean Cortical Width on Dental Panoramic Radiographs and thus diagnose women with low BMD or osteoporosis. • The accuracy, sensitivity, and specificity was93.0% (88.0%-98.0%), 95.8% (91.9%-99.7%)and86.6%(79.9%-93.3%),respectively on basis of the lumbar spine BMD; and 89.0%(82.9%-95.1%),96.0%(92.2%-99.8%) and 84.0%(76.8%-91.2%),on basis of the femoral neck BMD.
Kavithaet al[62]	Hybrid Genetic Swarm Fuzzy(GSF)classifier	• The sensitivity, specificity and accuracy of the hybrid GSF with optimized Membership Function and Rule Set in identifying females with a low BMD were 95.3%, 94.7% and 96.01%, respectively, at the lumbar spine and 99.1%, 98.4% and 98.9%, respectively, at the femoral neck BMD
Hwangetal[63]	Decision Tree and Support vector machine (SVM)	• The endosteal margin area showed statistically significant differences in fractal dimension (FD), gray level co-occurrence matrix(GLCM), and 45 strut variables between the osteoporotic and non-osteoporotic patients, whereas the medullary 46 portions showed few distinguishing features. • The sensitivity, specificity,& accuracy of the strut 47 variables in the endosteal margin area were 97.1%, 95.7%, and 96.25 using the decision tree and 4897.2%, 97.1%, and 96.9% using SVM, and these were the best results obtained among the 3methods. 49 Strut variables with FD/GLCM didn't increase the diagnostic accuracy.

Table 3 Studies of the application of AI in the diagnosis of osteoporosis

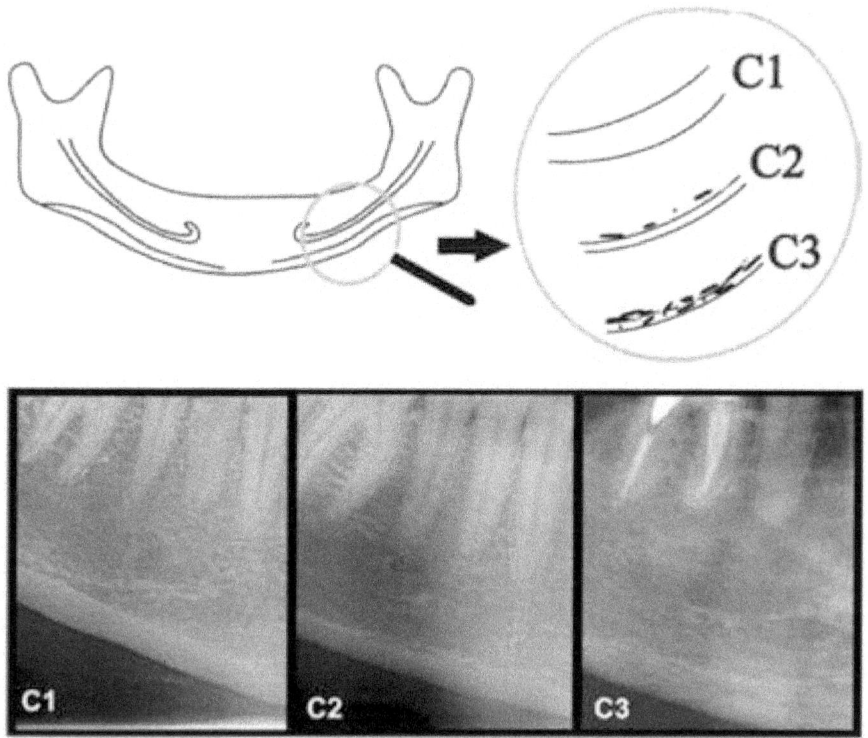

Figure 7 Representation of the Mandibular Cortical Index (MCI) according to Klemetti

(C1) normal cortex, when the endosteal margin of the cortex appears even and sharp on both sides;

(C2) moderately eroded cortex, when the endosteal margin shows semilunar defects (lacunar resorption) or appears to form endosteal cortical residue, and

(C3) severely eroded or porous cortex, when the cortical layers form dense endosteal cortical residue and are clearly porous

4.4 *Temporal mandibular Joint*

Jaw disorders can be divided into several subgroups. (64) One of them is temporomandibular joint disorders (TMDs) with noticeable signs like jaw joint noises, limitations in the opening of the jaw, difficulty in chewing (tiredness of jaw muscle), locking of the joint, ringing in the ear, neck pain & shoulder pain. TMD-related pain can affect the everyday routines mentally and physically of an individual, which in turn affects the quality of life. Internal derangements of the temporomandibular joint are yet another taxing situation where the expert examiners' decision based on clinical and imaging data is considered the gold standard. However, when trained ANNs were tested and compared with the diagnosis of a surgeon, the results revealed high sensitivity and specificity of ANN, thereby insisting on the importance of AI in achieving correct interpretations and reducing human errors. (65)

STUDY	TECHNIQUE	KEYFEATURES
Orhanet al [66]	**ML**	**o Radiomics platform was used to extract imaging features [first-order statistics, shape, texture, gray-level co-occurrence matrix(GLCM), gray-level run length matrix(GLRLM), and gray-level size zone matrix(GLSZM)] of TMJ pathologies, condylar bone changes, and disc displacement** **o Six classifiers, including logistic regression (LR), random forest(RF), decision tree(DT), k-nearest neighbors (KNN), XG Boost, and support vector machine (SVM) were used for model building** **o o k-nearest neighbor (KNN) and random forest (RF) classifiers were found to be the most optimal machine learning model to classify the condylar changes and TMJ disc displacements with AUC, sensitivity, and specificity for the training set were 0.89 and 1,while those for the testing set were 0.77 and 0.74, respectively, for condylar changes and disc displacement, respectively.**
Kim et al [67]	**R-CNN and CNN**	**o An algorithm to diagnose TMJ OA was designed. First, two algorithms were developed: one algorithm that detects the TMJ and surrounding anatomical structures (including joint fossa and condyle) and another algorithm that determines whether the detected anatomical region has any abnormality based on the shape of the TMJ. Finally, an algorithm to determine the presence or absence of TMJ OA was developed.** **o The average precision of condyle detection using an R-CNN at intersection over union (IoU) >0.5 is 99.4% (right side) and 100%(left side)** **o The sensitivity, specificity, and accuracy of the TMJ Osteoarthritis classification algorithm using a CNN are 0.54,0.94,and 0.84,respectively**

Table 4 Studies of the application of AI in diagnosing TMJ disorders

4.5 Muscles

Fast and accurate segmentation of musculoskeletal ultrasound images is an ongoing challenge. Two principal factors make this task difficult: firstly, the presence of speckle noise arising from the interference that accompanies all coherent imaging approaches; secondly, the sometimes subtle interaction between musculoskeletal components that leads to non-uniformity of the image intensity. CNN's are an effective tool that has previously been used in image processing of several biomedical imaging modalities.

STUDY	TECHNIQUE	KEY FEATURES
Jabbaret al[68]	**CNN**	o **Pixel-based edge-detection on Musculoskeletal Ultrasound Images** o **Performance of CNNs trained on Expert Ground Truth image data outperform CNN strained on Canny Ground Truth Images in defining edges of muscle**

Table 5 Study of the applications of AI in musculoskeletal disorders

4.6 Paranasal Sinuses

Paranasal sinuses (PNS) are prone to inflammation and infection. The mucus drainage is interrupted when the paranasal sinuses become blocked from secretions or a mass, causing sinusitis. Depending on the cause, sinusitis is treated with corticosteroids, decongestants, nasal irrigation, and hydration. Rarely is surgical intervention required to enhance drainage.

STUDY	TECHNIQUE	KEYFEATURES
Junget al [69]	**DL**	• **For segmentation the maxillary sinus into the maxillary bone, air, and lesion**

Table 6 Study of the application of AI in PNS lesions

4.7 Nerves

Cranial nerves I (olfactory), II (optic), and VIII (vestibulocochlear) are considered purely afferent. Cranial nerves III(oculomotor), IV(trochlear), VI(abducens), XI(spinal accessory), and XII (hypoglossal) are purely efferent. The remaining cranial nerves, V(trigeminal), VII (facial), IX (glossopharyngeal), and X (vagus), are functionally mixed(sensory and motor).

Damage to the cranial nerves, their tracts, or nuclei results in stereotypical dysfunctions. While this is the classical way of organizing and indexing cranial nerves, the scientific reality is more complex and is still debated in the academic realm, including the classification and identification of the routes of distinct cranial nerves fibers and the presence or absence of other less recognized structures, such as the terminal nerve, also called nerve null or cranial nerve zero.

STUDY ON TRIGEMINAL NEURALGIA	TECHNIQUE	KEYFEATURES
Limonadi et al.[70]	ANN	• designed and trained an artificial neural network (ANN) and as an initial feasibility assessment of such an ANN system's ability to recognize and correctly diagnose patients with different facial pain syndromes • predicted the correct diagnosis for 95 of 100 patients (95%), and prospectively determine a correct diagnosis of trigeminal neuralgia Type 1 with 84% sensitivity and 83% specificity in 43 new patients.

Table 7 Study on the application of AI in Trigeminal Neuralgia

4.8 Cyst And Tumors

Odontogenic cysts and tumors are mandibular and maxillary lesions that occur across all patient demographics across age, sex, race, and social-economic status, as altered remnants of dental development. They may be incidental findings from routine imaging in any office or found through workup for craniofacial surgery or injury. Many of these patients present with asymptomatic lesions, whereas others may be symptomatic. (71)

STUDY ON CYSTS	TECHNIQUE	KEY FEATURES
Mikulka et al. (72)	ML	◦ Assessment of classification of Jaw Bone Cysts and Necrosis by processing of Orthopantomograms ◦ results of fast automatized segmentation by the live-wire method and comparison of the obtained data with the results provided by other segmentation techniques ◦ In addition, comparison of various classifiers is done in this study, including the Decision Tree, Naive Bayes, Neural Network, k-NN, SVM, and LDA classification tools. Within this comparison, the highest degree of accuracy was attributed to the Decision Tree, Naïve Bayes, and Neural Network classifiers
Abdolali et al.	ML	◦ ground-truth data set consisting of cone beam CT images of 96 patients, belonging to three maxillofacial cyst categories: radicular cyst, dentigerous cyst and keratocystic odontogenic tumor is utilized ◦ At first, each cystic lesion is segmented with high accuracy ◦ Then, in the second and third steps, feature extraction and classification are performed. ◦ Contourlet and SPHARM coefficients are utilized as texture and shape features which are fed into the classifier ◦ Two different classifiers are used in this study, i.e. support vector machine and sparse discriminant analysis. ◦ Generally SPHARM coefficients are estimated by the iterative residual fitting (IRF) algorithm which is based on stepwise regression method. ◦ In order to improve the accuracy of IRF estimation, a method based on extra orthogonalization is employed to reduce linear dependency. ◦ Classification accuracy reported to be improved by atleast 8.94%with respect to conventional features
◦ Rana et al (73)	◦ software iPlan and Smartbrush	◦ Comparitive study of manual segmentation of mandibular odontogenic cysts and tumors with threshold-based segmentation using the software iPlan (Brainlab AG, Feldkirchen, Germany) as well as with segmentation using the Smartbrush (Smartbrush 2.0, Brainlab AG,Feldkirchen,Germany) ◦ These three methods were compared regarding usability, time expenditure and accuracy

Table 8 Studies on the application of AI in cystic lesions

4.9 Lymph Node Metastasis

Although most metastatic neck nodes arise from primary tumors of the head and neck, isolated, supraclavicular, and or inferior neck lymphadenopathy should alert the clinician to consider the likely possibility of a non-head and neck primary neoplasm. The most common remote primary tumors associated with neck lymph node metastases include cancers of the breast, lung, kidney, cervix, and testis. The lymphatic anatomy supports a predilection for metastases to left-sided lymph nodes. An accurate tissue diagnosis is critical, taken in context with clinical presentation. (74)

STUDY	TECHNIQUE	KEYFEATURES
Dohopolski et al. [75]	**CNN**	o **Prediction of Lymph Node Metastasis in Patients with Oropharyngeal Cancer** o **Two models were constructed with differing architectures AlexNet-like or UNET.** o **AlexNet-like's AUC was 0.93. Sensitivity, specificity, positive predictive value (PPV), and negative predictive value(NPV) were 0.60, 0.94, 0.71, and 0.91,respectively.** o **UNET's AUC was 0.91. sensitivity, specificity, PPV, and NPV were 0.70, 0.93 ,0.70, and 0.93,respectively.**
Ariji et al. [76]	**DL**	o **CT evaluation of extranodal extension of cervical lymphnode metastasis in patients with oral squamous cell carcinoma** o **Deep learning diagnostic performance in extranodal extension was significantly higher than that of radiologists with 81% specificity, 75.4% sensitivity, 78.2% accuracy and area under curve 0.80.**

Table 9 Studies on the application of AI on lymph node metastasis

4.10 OPMDS

Early detection of premalignant lesions is very important. Therefore, miscellaneous modalities such as oral cavity examination, supravital staining, oral cytology, and optical technologies including spectroscopy, fluorescence spectroscopy, elastic scattering (reflectance) spectroscopy, Raman spectroscopy, fluorescence imaging, optical coherence tomography, narrow-band imaging, and multimodal optical imaging may be used other. (77) The application of AI in OPMDs is summarized in the table below:

STUDY	TECHNIQUE	KEYFEATURES
Maghsoudi et al[78]	**ANN**	**◦ To evaluate diagnostic prediction of Lichen Planus, Leukoplakia and Oral Squamous Cell Carcinoma using ANN ◦ The four features which are common in these diseases intended for the diseases (white lesion, oral involvement, age, gender), are selected and encoded to the range of [0,1] and further entered into the system in the forms of parameters p1 to p4 and with specific codes. ◦ Superior performance of ANN based model was observed.**

Table 9 Study of the application of AI in OPMDs

4.11 Oral Cancer

Oral cancer is one of the most prevalent cancers with high mortality (79), and it is a significant public health issue. Late diagnosis and high death rates are attributes of cancer around the world. According to the 2015 statistics of the World Health Organization (WHO), cancer is the first or the second driving reason of death in almost 91 of 172 countries. The diagnosis and prediction of the reoccurrence of OC are challenging factors, as AI involves complex data on etiology and risk factors.

AI is an exceptionally fresh development with a significant prognostic power, which allows clinicians to select appropriate treatment modalities. AI holds an incredible guarantee to empower clinicians to make noteworthy choices depending on the immense amount of digitized data. AI has a preferred advantage over existing techniques for detecting OC. It is a versatile innovation and can acquire additional information at any time.

As the late-stage disease has a poor prognosis, early detection is important in OC patients. The data obtained from mobile phone technologies, medical imaging techniques, fluorescent images, exfoliative cytology, predictor variable, and depth of invasion can be used in AI learning tools, and OC can be diagnosed quickly with more accuracy. (80)Several studies have carried out early detection of the advanced stage of OC, and studies have reported that OC arises from different subsites of the oral cavity such as tongue, buccal mucosa, etc. This heterogeneity of oral malignant growth makes it difficult to be analyzed.

STUDY ON MOBILE PHONE TECHNOLOGIES	TECHNIQUE	KEY FEATURES
Song et al.[81]	o Android Smartphone Luxeon LED o CNN o Transfer learning	o To screen high-risk populations for oral cancer using smart phone-based intraoral dual-modality immuno-fluorescence imaging platform and classification of images obtained o To compare the performance of different CNN and transfer learning o Best performance with AFI-WLI: VGG-CNN-M o Accuracy:86.9 Sensitivity:85.0 Specificity:88.7
Welikala et al. [82]	CNN	o To detect and classify oral lesions in low risk and high risk, first in a phase of collection with bonding box annotations from clinicians and after classifying by deep learning o Identification image that containing lesion(test): Precision:84.77 Recall: 89.51 F1Score:87.07 o Identification imaging that required referral (test): Precision:67.1 Recall: 93.8 F1Score: 78.3 o Refer-low risk OPMD/cancer or high OPMD (test): Precision:26.4/14.7 Recall:43.9/56.0 F1Score:33/23.3
Shamim et al. [83]	DCNN	o In this study, application and evaluation of the efficacy of six deep convolutional neural network (DCNN) models using transfer learning is done, for identifying pre-cancerous tongue lesions directly using a small data set of clinically annotated photographic images to diagnose early signs of OCC. o DCNN model based on Vgg19 architecture was able to differentiate between benign and precancerous tongue lesions with a mean classification accuracy of 0.98, sensitivity 0.89 and specificity 0.97 o Additionally, the ResNet50 DCNN model was able to distinguish between five types of tongue lesions i.e. hairy tongue, fissured tongue, geographic tongue, strawberry tongue and oral hairy leukoplakia with a mean classification accuracy of 0.97.

Table 11 Studies on the application of AI in mobile phone technologies in oral cancer

STUDY ON MEDICAL IMAGING TECHNIQUE	TECHNIQUE	KEY FEATURES
Jeyaraj & Nadar [84]	DL	o To develop a DL algorithm for automated, computer-aided oral cancer detecting system by investigating patient hyper spectral images o OCvs. Benign Accuracy:91.4 Sensitivity:94 Specificity:91 o Partitioned CNN vs. expert oncologist Accuracy:94.5 Sensitivity:94 Specificity:98
Poedjiastoeti et al [85]	CNN	o for the detection of ameloblastomas and KCOTs o Ameloblastomas and KCOTs could be detected based on digital panoramic radiographic images using CNN with accuracy comparable to that of manual diagnosis by oral maxillaofacial specialists. o These results demonstrate that CNN may KCOTs in a substantially shorter time

Table 12 Study on the application of AI in medical imaging techniques in oral cancer

STUDY ON FLUORESCENCE IMAGING	TECHNIQUE	KEY FEATURES
van Staveren et al. (86)	CNN	◦ To apply an Artificial Network of autofluorescence spectra for classifying either homogeneous or non-homogeneous leukoplakia ◦ Abnormal vs. Normal//Homogeneous v/s Non-homogeneous ◦ Sensitivity: 86//73/64/100 Specificity:100//82/94/86
STUDY ON EXFOLIATIVE CYTOLOGY	**TECHNIQUE**	**KEY FEATURES**
McRae et al. (87)	◦ SVM ◦ Lasso logistic regression ◦ Training:PCA ◦ Validation:K-NN	◦ discriminated early and late disease with AUCs(95% CI) of 0.82 (0.77 to 0.87) and 0.93 (0.88 to0.97)

Table 13 Study on application of AI in fluorescence imaging and exfoliative cytology in oral cancer

STUDY ON GENE EXPRESSION PROFILING	TECHNIQUE	KEYFEATURES
Shams and Htike[88]	**ML TECHNIQUES** ◦ DNN ◦ SVM ◦ REGULARIZED ◦ LEAST SQUARES ◦ MULTI LAYER PERCEPTRON	◦ to predict the possibility of oral cancer development in OPL patients ◦ With gene expression profiling ◦ Fisher discriminate analysis was used to select relevant features from the gene expression array ◦ DNN Accuracy (%) 83.7 Sensitivity (%) Cancer development 84.3 Specificity(%) Cancer free 82.8 ◦ SVM Accuracy (%) 84.8 Sensitivity (%) Cancer development 86.2 Specificity(%) Cancer free 82.8 ◦ RLS Accuracy (%) 80.2 Sensitivity (%)Cancer development 82.3 Specificity(%) Cancer free 77.1 ◦ MLP Accuracy (%) 83.7 Sensitivity (%) Cancer development 86.2 Specificity (%) Cancer free 80

Table 14 Study on the application of AI on gene expression profiling in oral cancer

STUDY ON CLINICAL SIGNS AND HISTORY TAKING	TECHNIQUE	KEY FEATURES
Sharma et al. (89)	Probabilistic Neural Network and General Regression Neural Network	o Helpful to practitioners for the following decisions: (a) To diagnose the malignant patients and the type of malignancy on the basis of demographic information, clinical symptoms, medical and personal history, and gross examination. (b) To predict the stage and extent of oral cancer on the basis of symptoms which are confirmed with the help of relevant tests and investigations. (c) To predict the survivability of patients after appropriate treatments and follow-ups Accuracy 99.02% Sensitivity 99.35% Specificity98.01% Area under ROC curve 0.9974

Table 15 Study on application of AI on clinical signs and history taking in oral cancer

4.12 Pigmented Lesions

The identification of pigmented tissue within the oral cavity may present a diagnostic dilemma for the clinician. The manifestation of mucosal pigment is variable and can range from focal to diffuse macular coloration or from a small nodular growth to a large mass. (90)

STUDY	TECHNIQUE	KEY FEATURES
Phillips et al[91]	Deep Learning	◦ determine the accuracy of an artificial intelligence algorithm in identifying melanoma in dermoscopic images of lesions taken with smartphone and digital single-lens reflex(DSLR) cameras ◦ The algorithm achieved an AUROC of 90.1%(95%CI, 86.3%-94.0%) for biopsied lesions and 95.8% (95%CI, 94.1%-97.6%) for all lesions using iPhone6 images; an AUROC of 85.8%(95%CI, 81.0%-90.7%) for biopsied lesions and 93.8%(95%CI, 91.4%-96.2%) for all lesions using Galaxy S6 images; Andan AUROC of 86.9%(95%CI, 80.8%- 93.0%) for biopsied lesions and 91.8%(95%CI,87.5%-96.1%) for all Lesions using DSLR camera images.

Table 16 Study of the application of AI for Pigmented Lesions

4.13 Uvb Lesions

Recurrent aphthous ulceration is one such condition without a precise etiology, where clinical diagnosis is made only on the basis of recurrence and by the exclusion of other factors.

STUDY	TECHNIQUE	KEY FEATURES
NS Dar-Odeh et al.[37]	Neural Network	• data from 86 participants were used to construct and train a neural network to predict the factors appearing to be related to the occurrence of recurrent aphthous ulcers. • When this was further tested using untrained data of 10 participants the results revealed most accurate predictions such as gender, hemoglobin, serum Vitamin B12, serum ferritin, red cell folate, salivary candidal colony count, frequency of tooth brushing, and the number of fruits or vegetables consumed to be related to recurrent aphthous ulceration and appropriate for use as input data to construct ANNs.

Table 17 Study of the applications of AI in UVB lesions

4.14 Psycho somatic Disorders

According to the Global Burden of Disease Study in 1990 and 2010, the main causes of the fourth largest disease burden measured in disability-adjusted life years (DALYs) are mental and substance-use disorders, which are jointly considered to be the leading cause of lived-with disability worldwide. (92)

Bayesian model

In AI, the naïve Bayes classifier is a general term for a classification algorithm. The naïve Bayesian method is a classification method based on Bayes' theorem and characteristic condition independent hypothesis.

Recent studies have often employed Bayesian models to diagnose psychiatric disorders. For example, the Strüngmann Forum on Computational Psychiatry proposed using Bayesian inference to connect underlying causes (genetics and sociological phenomena), latent hypothesized theoretical constructs, and symptoms. Control systems that use machine learning have also been used to automate the delivery of neuromuscular blockade, and these systems have also incorporated forecasting of drug pharmacokinetics to further improve the control of infusions of paralytics.

Logistic regression

In statistics, logistic models (or logit models) are widely used statistical models, and LR is an important AI algorithm. Recent studies often employ LR models to diagnose psychiatric disorders. For example, Hagen et al. (93) evaluated the associations between psychological distress and two cognitive screening tools by means of an LR method. The results demonstrated that performance-based assessment could reduce the impact of psychological distress on cognitive screening.

In addition, Barker et al. (94) employed models of multivariable LR to predict 30-day psychiatric readmission. Their findings are considered to be crucial predictors for psychiatric readmission and have provided a better way of readmission prediction. Shen et al. (95) generated a risk stratification model to obtain the odds ratio (OR) of psychiatric comorbidities by a classification and regression tree method. Using the LR method, the odds ratio of psychiatric comorbidities was calculated between subjects with and without borderline personality disorder. In general, the accuracy of LR models is so high that they are commonly applied in clinical practice.

Decision tree

A decision tree is a flowchart-like diagram (Figure 8) that shows the various outcomes from a series of decisions, including chance event outcomes and utility. Decision trees are one of the most widely and broadly used algorithms for supervised classification learning. In AI, a decision tree is a predictive model that represents a mapping between object properties and object values. Most modern decision tree learning algorithms adopt a purity-based heuristic. Carpenter et al. (96) used the decision tree algorithm to test whether an individual Preschool Age Psychiatric Assessment (PAPA) item can predict whether a child is likely to have a generalized anxiety disorder (GAD) or separation anxiety disorder (SAD).

They used a decision tree to identify children who were on the brink of experiencing an anxiety disorder, and their results showed that the decision tree could achieve accurate prediction up to 96% for both GAD and SAD. With a decision tree, Sattler et al. (97) analyzed data from the Spence Children's Anxiety Scale (SCAS) and SCAS-Pobsessive–compulsive disorder subscales, and worked out two screening algorithms to diagnose obsessive–compulsive disorder from a combined clinical and community sample of children and families. The results showed that the algorithms that reduced the number of SCAS-P items needed to make a diagnosis of obsessive–compulsive disorder diagnoses up to 67%–83% without sacrificing the nature relative to the full subscales.

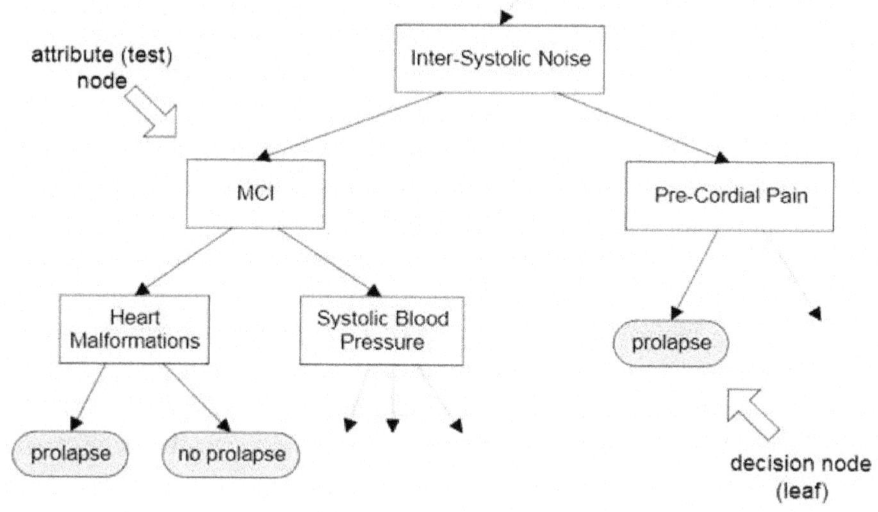

Figure 8 Example of Decision Tree

Support vector machines

The SVM is a current supervised learning method, the decision boundary of which is the maximum margin hyperplane for solving learning samples. SVM models have been commonly used for diagnosing psychiatric disorders. For example, in order to describe users' situations. Peng et al. (98) employed a multi-kernel SVM-based model to locate potential users who might suffer from depression by extracting three social methods (user microblog text, user profile, and user behaviors). Based on a multiclass

SVM, Al-Shargie et al. (94) put forward a discriminant analysis method. The results showed that the method could discriminate between different stress levels for EE with a 94.79% average classification accuracy.

Deep Learning

Classic machine learning methods, such as the Bayesian model and SVM, have been widely employed in psychiatry and neuroscience studies for a long time. At present, deep learning, which is a hot machine learning research direction, outperforms the aforementioned AI models by a considerable margin.

Deep learning refers to a set of algorithms on a multi-layer neural network that uses various machine learning algorithms to solve various problems such as images and text. Combined with low-level features, deep learning can develop more abstract high-level attribute categories or features that can discover distributed feature representations of data. By leveraging DNNs on the tensor Flow framework, Khan et al. (88) proposed a computational tool (integrated mental-disorder Genome score, or iMEGES) to analyze the whole genome/exome sequencing data on personal genomes.

Based on the deep learning framework, this tool creates prioritized gene scores for psychiatric disorders. The findings revealed that the property of this tool is better than that of competing approaches when a large training dataset is available.

In addition, Heinsfeld et al.(99) applied deep learning algorithms on a large brain imaging dataset in order to identify patients with autism spectrum disorder based solely on the patients' brain activation patterns. The findings revealed that 70% accuracy was achieved in the dataset and that the deep learning method scan classifies large datasets better than other methods.

Furthermore, the results showed the promise of deep learning for clinical datasets and illustrated the future application of AI in the identification of mental disorders. Although extremely advanced performance has been demonstrated in several fields, deep learning has been under close concern for its lack of transparency during the learning and testing processes. For example, deep learning has been referred to as a "blackbox." In comparison, techniques such as LR are simple and easy to understand.

4.15 Anesthesiology

Artificial intelligence has been advancing in fields including anesthesiology. The six themes of applications of artificial intelligence in anesthesiology:
(1) Depth of anesthesia monitoring
(2) Control of anesthesia
(3) Event and risk prediction
(4) Ultrasound guidance
(5) Pain management
(6) Operating room logistics. (100)

Kendale et al.conducted a supervised learning study on electronic health record data with the goal of identifying patients who experienced post-induction hypotension (mean arterial pressure [MAP] less than 55 mmHg). The training dataset included 70% of the patients and variables such as the American Society of Anesthesiologists (ASA) physical status, age, body mass index, comorbidities, and medications, as well as the blood pressure of the patients. The various algorithms used by Kendale et al. could then analyze the training dataset to learn which variables were predictive of post-induction hypotension. The test dataset was then analyzed to assess how accurately the algorithm could predict post-induction hypotension in the remaining 30% of patients.

Unsupervised learning refers to algorithms identifying patterns or structures within a dataset. This can be useful for finding novel ways of classifying patients, drugs, or other groups. Begin et al. used unsupervised learning techniques to mine data from the Food and Drug Administration drug labels to identify the major topics (e.g., specific adverse events, therapeutic application) into which drugs could be automatically classified for hypothesis generation for future research.

Reinforcement Learning refers to the process by which an algorithm is asked to attempt a certain task (e.g., deliver inhalational anesthesia to a patient, or drive a car) and to learn from its subsequent mistakes and successes. A biological analogy to reinforcement learning is operant conditioning, where the classical example is of a rat taught to push a lever through the use of a food-based reward. However, reinforcement learning problems today are more sophisticated. For example, Padmanabhan et al. used reinforcement learning to develop an anesthesia controller that used feedback from a patient's bispectral index(BIS) and MAP to control the infusion rates of Propofol (in a simulated patient model). In this scenario, achieving BIS and MAP values within a set range results in a reward to the algorithm, whereas values outside the range result in errors that prompt the algorithm to perform further fine-tuning.

Machine learning problems are often divided into those that require classification (dividing data into discrete groups) and those that require regression (modeling data to better understand the relationship between two or more continuous variables with the potential for prediction). A frequent example of classification is image recognition (e.g., recognizing a cat vs. a dog), whereas a frequent example of regression is prediction (e.g., predicting house prices from preexisting data on square footage).

Fuzzy logic often uses rule-based systems (e.g., if...then systems) that have been largely used in control systems where precise mathematical functions do not accurately model phenomena. For example, an anesthesia monitor to detect hypovolemia was developed using fuzzy logic to approximate the presence of mild, moderate, and severe hypovolemia based on normalized values of heart rate (HR), blood pressure, and pulse volume that was divided into categories of mild, moderate, and severe. The monitor used rules built on fuzzy logic such as "If (electrocardiogram-HR is mild) and (blood pressure is mild) and (pulse volume is severe), then (hypovolemia is moderate)".

The development of such rules requires expert human input to determine an appropriate rule set for the machine to follow, and early studies in fuzzy logic and other adaptive control mechanisms help set the foundation for exploring more modern approaches to imprecise information or incomplete data. More recent research in the field has used artificial intelligence approaches to better evaluate and use data to trigger the rule functions of fuzzy systems. Thus, although research in fuzzy logic systems is ongoing (especially in control systems for applications such as medication delivery), progress in artificial intelligence research has focused on using more data-driven techniques in machine learning to achieve goals first explored by researchers working with fuzzy logic.

Machine learning uses features, or properties within the data, to perform its tasks. To analogize an example in statistical analysis, features would be analogous to independent variables in logistic regression. In classical machine learning, the features are selected (often referred to as hand-crafted) by experts to help guide the algorithms in the analysis of complex data. Decision tree learning is a type of supervised learning algorithm that can be used to perform either classification (classification trees) or regression tasks (regression trees). As its name implies, this set of techniques uses flowchart-like tree models with multiple branch points to determine a target value or classification from an input. Each node within a tree has an assigned value, and the final node represents an endpoint and the cumulative probability of arriving at that point based on the preceding decisions. Hu et al. used decision trees to predict total patient-controlled analgesia (PCA) consumption from features such as patient demographics, vital signs, and aspects of their medical history, surgery type, and PCA doses delivered with the promise of using such approaches to optimize PCA dosing regimens. The k-nearest neighbor algorithms area group of supervised learning algorithms that assesses training data geometrically and then determine whether additional input data falls into a category based on the training examples plotted nearest to it (based on Euclidian distance). Based on the specific approach used, this may be based on a single nearest point (1-nearest neighbor) or the weight of a group of points (k-nearest neighbor). Support vector machines are another type of supervised learning algorithm that can also be used for both classification and regression. Support vector machines map training data in space and then use hyperplanes to optimally separate the data into representative categories or clusters. New data are then classified based on their location in space relative to the hyperplane.

One of the most popular methods today for performing work in machine learning is the use of neural networks. Neural networks are inspired by biological nervous systems and process signals in layers of computational units (neurons). Each network is made up of an input layer of neurons comprised of features that describe the data, at least one hidden layer of neurons that conduct different mathematical transformations on the input features, and an output layer that yields a result (fig. 4). Between each layer are multiple connections between neurons that are parameterized to different weights depending on the input-output maps. Thus, neural networks are a framework within which different machine learning algorithms can work to achieve a particular task (e.g., image recognition, data classification). Modern neural network architecture has expanded to allow for deep learning, neural networks that use many layers to learn more complex patterns than those that are discernible from simple one- or two-layer networks. Subtypes of deep learning networks that one may encounter are convolutional neural networks, which can process data composed of multiple arrays, and recurrent neural networks, which are better designed to analyze sequential data (e.g., speech).

CHAPTER FIVE

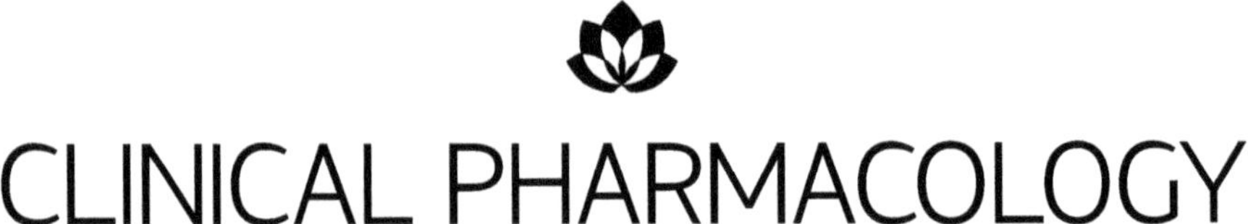

CLINICAL PHARMACOLOGY

"Predicting the future isn't magic; it's artificial intelligence."
-Dave Waters

5.1 Introduction

In modern drug discovery (101), creating the molecule libraries, identifying novel drug candidates with optimal properties, predicting the biological functions of proteins, and deep learning play critical roles. In the early phase of drug discovery, the elimination of inactive or toxic compounds is of critical significance. Machine learning classification methods (Table 2) have been applied for screening and classification of drugs or non-drug collections and prediction of toxicities. Moreover, machine learning methods help to model the metabolism of drugs, including their interactions with metabolic enzymes or relationships between the chemical structures of drugs and their biological fates and metabolic endpoints that may result in more accurate prediction of metabolic fates and potential toxicities of new drug candidates.

CLASSIFICATION METHODS	APPLICATIONS
Support vector machines	• **Prediction of the activity of enzyme inhibitors or rate-limited drug absorption** • **Example: In a QSAR study, 1,4 dihydro-pyridine calcium channel antagonists have been screened by least square support vector machine**
Supervised learning algorithms	• **Prediction of drug-target interactions** • **Example: regularized least squares classifier for prediction of drug-target interactions** • **Remark: Semi-supervised link prediction classifier has shown high performance in predicting drug target interactions**
Combination of Gaussian interaction profile kernels and genomic and chemical kernels	• **Better predictive power**

Table 18 Application of Machine learning in pharmacology

Using ANNs

It would be possible to model the complex biological data and non-linear systems, solve the problems of multivariate and multi-response systems, predict the secondary structures of proteins, apply for detection of amino acids with similar structures, and determine concentrations of chiral samples or enantiomeric excess modeling the reaction rates such as the conversion rates of the oxidation reaction and prediction of the behavior of semi-batch reactors in a series of experimental conditions automated algorithm for evaluation of the metabolic transformations of compounds in order to classify drug candidates as substrates of cytochrome P-450 evaluation of the organ-targeting peptides which were selected from a random phage-peptide library using phage display technique Drug loading, saturation solubility, and diffusion coefficient were predicted with a relative error of 1%. The development of deep neural network models provides the possibility to predict the pharmacological profiles of drugs, including their mechanisms of action and indications.

AI approaches may also be applied to develop

- The predictive models
- Identify the biomarkers
- Construct correlations between the gene expression profile and clinical phenotype
- Facilitate the personalized therapies
- Rapid identification of the bioactive molecules among millions of compounds. Example: For quantification of two forms of ranitidine-HCl, ANNs have enabled rapid identification of the form1 in a multi-component tablet.
- Optimizing drug release from matrix tablets. Example: Making a correlation between the formulation factors and release profiles.
- Besides the prediction of dissolution and release profiles, ANNs are useful for optimizing modified-release products, including solid dosage forms.
- Assessment of the kinetic curves and data parameters in the chemical reaction.

5.2 Correlation between the formulation factors and release profiles using AI

ANNs are useful for optimizing modified-release products, including solid dosage forms. GRNNs and connectionist models help to predict drug stability and release profiles. Using ANNs, a semi-empirical mathematical model capable of predicting the released drug amount from solid lipid extrudates has been developed. System inputs included the diameter and length of the extrudates and dissolution times, and the amount of released diprophylline was considered as output. Using the modified Weibull equation, it has been revealed that enhancement of the extrudate diameter results in a reduced release rate. ANNs have also been used to design the optimal formulations of sustained release dosage forms and predict their dissolution profiles. GRNN has been applied for designing the extended-release aspirin tablets. In order to obtain optimal aspirin tablets, an optimized GRNN model has been applied for the prediction of formulation characteristics and process factors.

Based on the difference and similarity factors (f1 and f2), there was no difference between GRNN- predicted and experimentally-observed drug release profiles indicating the suitability of GRNN for modeling extended-release tablets. Using MLP neural network and backpropagation algorithm, diclofenac sodium extended-release tablets have been optimized. The amounts of Carbopol® 71G and Kollidon® K-25 were selected as network inputs, and in vitro dissolution time profiles were considered as outputs. Calculated similarity and difference factors revealed no difference between the experimental and predicted drug release profiles indicating the suitability of MLP for the prediction of drug release and its applicability for modeling and optimizing sustained-release tablet formulations. Dynamic neural networks capable of modeling dissolution profiles and more precise prediction of drug release profiles (as compared to MLP and static networks) have been applied for modeling the release of diclofenac sodium from polyethylene oxide controlled release matrix tablets. Networks with different topologies were established to obtain an accurate prediction of release profiles from the test formulations. Compression force and polymer fraction were demonstrated as the most dominant factors in the drug release profile. Furthermore, polyethylene oxides with high molecular weights proved to be more suitable for the development of controlled release dosage forms.

Similarity and difference factors demonstrated the ability of dynamic networks for accurate predictions. GRNN has been applied for the development of a multi-unit particulate system for controlled delivery of diclofenac sodium, modeling the effects of causal factors on the release profile of the drug from compressed matrix pellets and obtaining the optimal formulation. Correlation plots of the obtained and predicted values of drug release demonstrated the suitability of the GRNN model (R2 ~ 0.98). Furthermore, the percentage of the polymer was recognized as the controlling factor of drug release from the compressed matrix pellets. A combination of RSM and ANN methods has been used to optimize the formulation of isradipine-contained osmotic tablets. The difference between the predicted and observed dissolution profiles of the optimized formulation was within the experimental error limits. Furthermore, calculated similarity and difference factors revealed no difference between the predicted and experimental drug release profiles, indicating the suitability of ANN models for obtaining suitable dissolution profiles and developing controlled release formulations. For optimizing salbutamol sulfate osmotic pump tablets, an ANN model has been developed in which the causal factors included the amounts of hydroxyl propyl methyl cellulose, polyethylene glycol 1500 in the coating solution, and coat weight. The average drug release rate and correlation coefficient of the amount of drug released was considered as the response variables. Using a trained ANN model, optimal formulation factors were acquired. Following the preparation and in vitro test of the optimized formulation, the release rate and correlation coefficient of the optimized formulation showed a good agreement with the predicted effects. ANN and design expert systems have been applied for preparing glipizide push-pull osmotic pump tablets. Besides performing dissolution testing, the range of formulation factors and procedures was optimized by ANN. ANNs have also been employed to optimize nimodipine zero-order release matrix tablet formulation. For all responses, feed forward back propagation ANN demonstrated a better fit than multiple linear regression (MLR) models. Furthermore, the estimation of the similarity factor confirmed the ability of ANNs to increase prediction efficiency. In order to improve the accuracy of ANN models in the pharmaceutical research area, software for parameter optimization has been developed, which enables the estimation of suitable ANN parameters that might be of great significance for the development of optimal formulations, including sustained release tablets. The short half-life of melatonin, an effective agent against sleep disorders, necessitates the development of extended-release tablets. Meanwhile, mimicking the plasma levels of melatonin appears quite challenging. An ANN model has been applied to optimize melatonin release from hydrophilic polymer matrices. The model proved to be useful for optimizing the composition of extended-release melatonin tablets with suitable dissolution profiles.

ANN models have also been employed to predict the response variables, release parameters, and plasma concentrations of theophylline tablets. Findings demonstrated a good agreement between ANN-predicted and experimental values. Using ANNs, a comparative analysis of the release profiles and mucoadhesive of buccal tablets of propranolol hydrochloride was performed, and the polymers for the optimized formulation were identified. For obtaining increased mucoadhesion, polymers were selected by screening procedure and application of feed-forward back propagation ANN model. MLP network accurately identified the most significant input variables and suitable polymers for optimizing multi-polymeric propranolol buccal tablets. PEG exhibited the most significant effect on the mucoadhesive and mean dissolution time. MSE of 0.002 demonstrated the high efficiency of the trained model, and comprehensive knowledge was obtained about the behavior of polymeric matrix tablets that might be helpful for optimizing multi-polymer drug delivery systems.

Beads, pellets, and microspheres

Several ANN models have also been developed to predict dissolution profiles of controlled release particulates, including the beads, pellets, and microspheres. A model constructed by CAD/CAM software has been applied for modeling the effects of formulation variables and processes on the release profile of verapamil from the multi-particulate beads. Drug release data of the optimized formulations were in good agreement with those predicted by the ANN model.

An ANN model has been used for the assessment of the impact of process parameters on the entrapment of papain in cross-linked alginate beads leading to improved stability and site-specific delivery. Using optimal conditions, the neural network was constructed for the prediction of the experimental matrix. Dissolution studies in the pH range similar to those in the human gastrointestinal tract showed that alginate beads can be applied for delivery of papain to the small intestine. Accelerated and long-term stability evaluations revealed a significant improvement in the shelf-life of papain entrapped in alginate beads, indicating the usefulness of the method for the development of stable beads capable of site-specific drug delivery. ANNs provide useful information about the pellet properties and identify the relationships between the formulation characteristics, pelletization mechanisms, and key process variables. Using neuro-fuzzy systems for the prediction of the aspect ratio of pellets and characterizing preparation parameters might be a promising approach for further formulation procedures. Using MLP neural network, the dissolution profile of matrix-controlled release theophylline pellets has been predicted. Regarding the granulated pellet-containing tablets, pellet size, Eudragit FS 30D, hardness of tablets, and coating weight gain have been identified as influential factors for the evaluation of tablet properties, including the release behavior. High correlation coefficients between ANN predicted and experimental values demonstrated the suitable prediction power of ANNs. Aspirin-loaded calcium alginate floating microspheres have been optimized by ANNs and RSM in which the amounts of formulation materials and release and floating rate of microspheres were used as inputs and outputs, respectively. As compared to RSM, ANNs more accurately predicted in vitro drug release profiles. In the formulation of verapamil hydrochloride-loaded polymer microspheres, the pH of the external aqueous phase has been shown as the major determinant of incorporation efficiency and drug release behavior. ANN and factorial analysis as multi-variate methods were applied to assess the impact of combined effects of external phase pH and other parameters, initial drug loading, and polymer concentration on the properties of polymer microspheres. Besides better fitting abilities, the ANN model demonstrated less biased and more precise predictability than factorial analysis. In this context, ANN models have been successfully applied for multivariate modeling of the release or encapsulation of ionizable drugs from hydrophobic polymer microspheres.

For the preparation of the acrylic microspheres for controlled drug release, an ANN model has been developed for the evaluation of the effects of preparative variables during the solvent evaporation method. Input variables included the ratio of polymers, stirring rate, and concentration of the dispersing agent. The size of the microspheres and T63.2% were selected as response variables. ANN model showed higher predictability than MLR, suggesting that for evaluation of the formulation and process parameters, ANN models are suitable alternatives to the conventional regression methods.

Solid dispersions

Preparation of the solid dispersions is a promising approach to the improvement of drug solubility. A combination of ANNs and mixture experimental design has been applied for the development of solid dispersions. To improve the dissolution rate of carbamazepine, carbamazepine-Soluplus®-poloxamer188 solid dispersions were prepared by solvent casting method. The effect of solid dispersion composition on the dissolution rate of carbamazepine was assessed by three layers feed-forward MLP network and mixture experimental design. The relationship between the components of solid dispersion and the percentage of the released drug was well described by the mixture experimental design and ANN model; meanwhile, the MLP network demonstrated better predictability than the mixture experimental design. For the preparation of PVP/PEG mixtures as carriers for the development of drug solid dispersions, a feed forward back propagation ANN with logistic sigmoid activation function has been applied to make the correlation between the factors and dissolution characteristics and optimize dissolution rate. ANNs demonstrated suitable prediction power, and the prepared solid dispersions showed long-term physical stability. Nimodipine-PEG solid dispersion has been used for the development of effervescent controlled-release floating tablet formulations. A combination of experimental design and machine learning algorithms, including genetic programming and ANN, demonstrated suitable prediction power during the optimization process. Furthermore, simultaneous erosion and swelling were identified as the major mechanisms of the release of active ingredients.

Implants

For the management of the postsurgical problems associated with cochlear implantation, coating of the cochlear implants has been suggested for topical delivery of drugs against inflammation or infections. An ANN model has been applied for the prediction of the formulation parameters and release profile of dexamethasone from the cochlear implant coatings. For obtaining an appropriate drug release profile, the ability of the ANN model to determine the optimal levels of formulation parameters was evaluated. Besides providing a shorter formulation design process, the drug release profile from the implant device was accurately modeled by the ANN model, and the results were so close to the experimentally obtained values indicating the model's effectiveness.

Liposomes

Over the last decade, the application of echogenic liposomes for the delivery of chemotherapeutics has attracted growing interest. Since multiple drug resistance can be overcome by controlled drug release, an ANN-based model predictive controller has been proposed for constant release of the chemotherapeutic agent and maintaining an appropriate concentration at the tumor site that may reduce the risk of multi-drug resistance and short treatment duration. In order to design and optimize formulation parameters of leuprolide acetate-loaded liposomes, ANNs and MLR methods have been compared. To determine optimal ANN structure, various training sessions were carried out with different numbers of nodes in the hidden layer. Nonlinear differential transfer functions were applied to predict the percentage of drug entrapment in liposomal formulations. Based on the findings, the application of the feed forward back propagation network and MLR is a promising approach for predicting appropriate composition for a specific response and acquiring a piece of deeper knowledge about the effects of formulation parameters and preparation process on the product properties. A comparison of the predicted and experimental data revealed no statistically significant difference. Furthermore, optimal ANN showed higher predictive power than the MLR method because of the lower values of normalized error and higher precision level.

Transdermal formulations

An ANN model has been developed for optimizing transdermal ketoprofen hydrogel. Optimal values of the response variables were applied for optimizing gel composition. The results obtained from the optimal formulation showed a suitable agreement with those predicted by the ANN model. For transdermal delivery of melatonin, ANNs and RSM have been applied to optimize the vehicle composition. The transdermal route was selected to prevent the remarkable hepato-gastrointestinal first-pass metabolism of melatonin and maintain its steady-state plasma concentrations for appropriate time periods. Since melatonin is unable to pass through the dense lipophilic matrix of the stratum corneum, several solvents and their mixtures were used for enhancement of melatonin flux and reduction of lag time. A multilayer feed-forward back propagation network was developed for identifying the best solvent mixtures for a particular response and assessment of the inter-relativity between the responses. A multilayer feed-forward back propagation network was developed for identifying the best solvent mixtures for a particular response and assessment of the inter-relativity between the responses. Multi-layer feed-forward back propagation network was developed for identifying the best solvent mixtures for a particular response and assessment of the inter-relativity between the responses.

Regarding the potential of a neural network-based intelligent learning system for the prediction of the release profiles of drugs, an experimental study regarding transdermal iontophoresis has been conducted to assess the usefulness of a neural network model, Gaussian mixture model (GMM), for modeling and prediction of drug release profiles.

Using the face-centered central composite design (CCD) approach, several tests were systematically designed for simultaneous evaluation of the effects of process variables during iontophoresis. A combination of GMM and face-centered CCD has been suggested as a useful intelligent learning system for the prediction of the release profiles of drugs.

Hydrodynamically balanced systems, suppositories, pulmonary delivery

ANNs have been applied as modeling tools for predicting the release profiles of drugs from hydrodynamically balanced systems. Based on the chemical structure of drugs and formulation description, ANNs helped to accurately predict the release profiles of various drugs and identify the key variables affecting drug release. An ANN approach, along with modeling and simulation of the compartment-based models, has been applied for the assessment of differences between the slower and faster release of paracetamol from the layered excipient suppositories. It has been revealed that the extent of drug absorption is enhanced by the absorption increasing the effect of mono-di-glycerides and liver bypass mechanism. For designing the pulmonary drug delivery systems, two-layer perceptron feed-forward back propagation ANNs have been successfully used for simulating aerosol behavior.

Controlled-release formulations

The application of ANNs and fuzzy logic algorithm for designing of sustained release formulations helps to analyze the effects of formulation components on the release characteristics and optimize drug formulations. In this context, controlled release formulations of clopidogrel have been developed using a fuzzy logic algorithm and ANN analysis for determining the effects of tablet components on the release characteristics. Following the development of complex dosage forms and designing controlled-release formulations by pharmacokinetics simulations and ANNs, a good agreement has been found between the experimental findings and ANNs-based predictions. Based on the content of separate components in colloidal delivery systems and the nature of co-surfactants, GAs and ANNs can be used to predict the phase behavior of this type of delivery system. GA and supervised ANN have been used for selecting the key molecular descriptors and making correlations between the selected descriptors and the weight ratio of the system components and phase behavior, respectively. Findings have shown the influential role of the chemical compositions, molecular volume, lipophilic-hydrophilic balance, length of the hydrocarbon chain, and hydrocarbon volume of co-surfactants. The genetic neural network model predicted the phase behavior of the colloidal delivery systems with high accuracy, suggesting the suitability of this approach for the evaluation of the co-surfactants in pharmaceutical formulations.

Emulsions

Appropriate preparation of the emulsions necessitates a high level of expertise and technical knowledge. Based on the limitations of RSM, including the poor estimation of the optimal emulsions, ANNs capable of optimizing and modeling the complex relationships between the formulation parameters and their effects on the quality of the final product have been applied for the preparation of stable emulsions. In a study conducted by Kumar et al., ANNs have been used for formulating stable oil-in-water emulsions and optimizing the concentration of fatty alcohol. Input data included the variables of lauryl alcohol concentrations and time, and zeta potential, particle size, viscosity, and conductance were considered as outputs. Based on the validation experiments, ANN-predicted values were in good agreement with experimental data. ANNs have also shown promising accuracy in the prediction of the microemulsion type from its composition. Using the combination of evolutionary ANNs and GA, internal structures and types of microemulsions have been predicted with high accuracy. An ANN model has been developed to predict stable microemulsion formulation containing isoniazid and rifampicin for oral delivery. Data from several pseudo ternary phase triangles containing the mixture of surfactants and oil components were applied for training, testing, and validation of the ANN model. Using the radial basis function network architecture, weight ratios of the individual components were consistent with observed phase behavior. The obtained microemulsion formulation with improved stability was capable of targeted delivery of both anti-tuberculous drugs during the continuation phase suggesting the formulation's effectiveness in overcoming the problems associated with the combination of drugs with different solubilities.

Microparticles

In order to overcome the dissolution rate-limiting step, benznidazole chitosan microparticles have been prepared by the coacervation method, followed by the application of an ANN model for optimizing the formulation. Multi-response optimization was applied to obtain the maximal yield, encapsulation efficiency, and dissolution rate, and minimal size. ANN-predicted optimum values were in agreement with experimental findings indicating the appropriateness of ANNs for the development of the optimal benznidazole chitosan microparticles. Using ANNs capable of being trained online, an adaptive drug delivery system has been developed for more efficient treatment of infectious diseases.

Nanomaterials

Evaluation of the parameters which affect nanoparticle size, loading efficiency, or cytotoxicity might be helpful for designing more efficient drug delivery systems.ANNs have been applied to predict the physicochemical properties of nanoparticles with theranostic importance against a variety of disorders, analyze complex nonlinear relationships and factors affecting the stability or size of nanoparticles, or design the models for identifying the relationships between the factors affecting the development of controlled-release drug delivery systems.

Besides demonstrating input-output interactions, ANNs can be used for modeling and identification of key parameters which affect the size of nanoparticles in a multidimensional space. For the preparation of the biodegradable nanoparticles of tri-block poly(lactide)–poly(ethylene glycol)–poly (lactide) (PLA–PEG–PLA) copolymers drug carrier, an ANN model has been developed for identifying the factors affecting the nanoparticle size. Three-layer feed forward back propagation ANN was applied for modeling the preparation of nanoparticles, and the best predictive model was selected based on the appropriate R2 and MSE values for training, test, and validation data. Among the processing factors, polymer concentration was found to be the most influencing factor. For optimizing the formulation of polymer-lipid hybrid nanoparticles for controlled delivery of verapamil hydrochloride and assessment of the effects of formulation factors, optimization and modeling were performed based on the spherical central composite design. Multi-objective optimization of nanoparticles was performed using the validated ANN models and continuous GAs. The obtained nanoparticles showed suitable properties such as drug loading efficiency of 92% and mean particle size of 100 nm, which are desirable for lymphatic transport after oral administration. Predicted response variables were in good agreement with experimental findings. Comparing the predictive performance of ANN models and RSM revealed the better generalization and recognition ability of ANNs. Combining factorial design, ANN, and continuous GAs is a promising approach for multi-objective optimization and modeling of nanoformulations with suitable properties. Using ANN, formulation parameters of chitosan-tripolyphosphate nanoparticles have been optimized in order to control nanoparticle size and improve the process yield at a novel pH. Multilayer feed-forward back-propagation neural network was applied for modeling the complex nonlinear relationship between the inputs and outputs and presenting outputs as 3D graphs. ANN architecture included three layers, and a trial and error approach was carried out for modeling. Various training parameters were used for obtaining an appropriate predictive network, and two approaches were applied to prevent over-training of the network. The concentration of sodium tri-polyphosphate was found to have the greatest impact on the particle size and yield. Furthermore, the successful interaction of chitosan and sodium 2q nanoparticle formation was confirmed by differential scanning calorimetry and Fourier transform infrared spectroscopy indicating the ability of ANNs to predict the size and yield of nano-particles and identification of the influential factors. In this respect, the multivariate trained model capable of providing a deeper knowledge about the parameters affecting the physicochemical properties of nano-particles and predicting or optimizing the processing conditions are promising tools for obtaining improved diagnostic outcomes. Regarding the albumin-loaded chitosan nanoparticles prepared by the polyelectrolyte complexation technique, ANNs have been applied for the simultaneous determination of the effects of independent variables on dependent ones. Based on the findings, material concentrations are the most important factors affecting dependent variables, i.e., loading efficiency and cytotoxicity. In this sense, optimizing independent variables is necessary for obtaining suitable nanoparticles.

ANN models have also been applied for constructing a correlation between the entrapment efficiency of solid lipid or polymeric nano-particles and the prediction of the binding energy of drugs. In order to overcome the problems associated with the application of nano-emulsions, ANNs have been applied for modeling the experimentally obtained data, evaluating the factors which affect the cytotoxicity of nano-emulsion, and obtaining stable nano-emulsion systems with reduced cytotoxicity. Based on model findings, and surfactant and oil concentrations are the dominant factors affecting nanoemulsion stability and cytotoxicity, respectively. In this context, ANNs have been shown as promising tools for describing the effects of nanoemulsion ingredients on stability and cell viability. ANN models are also helpful for the identification of the key factors affecting the particle size of Nanoemulsions. An ANN model capable of modeling the formulation and processing experimental data related to budesonide nanoemulsion has identified the parameters which affect the particle size. The total amount of energy used during the nanoemulsion preparation was recognized as the main factor affecting the particle size of the nanoemulsion. Because of the multi-variate nature, the development of drug-loaded nanospheres is an expensive and time-consuming process. ANN and GA have been used to simulate and optimize the fabrication process of agar nanospheres. GA and ANN proved to be more efficient tools than RSM for modeling and optimizing the manufacturing process of bupropion-loaded agar nanospheres and estimating their physicochemical properties. In designing efficient nanoformulations, controlled release profiles and targeted delivery are the essential factors that should be taken into account. In this sense, designing the functional and specific linkers which affect the stability, release profile, and efficiency of nanotherapeutics might be of critical importance. Application of advanced linker technologies, including simulation and modeling techniques, web-based systems, GAs, or GA/fuzzy hybrid algorithms, helps to identify suitable linker candidates and develop novel linker-drug conjugates with enhanced efficiency and reduced toxicity.

Using ANNs, the formulation of the nano-particulate fingolimod delivery system has been optimized. The amounts of polyvinyl alcohol, poly (3-hydroxybutyrate-co-3-hydroxy valerate), fingolimod, and time of drug release have been considered as input values. Output data included the polydispersity index, particle size, entrapment efficacy, loading capacity, and percentage of drug release from nanoparticles. Feed forward back propagation was applied to assess the effect of time on the percentage of drug release, and the optimal formulation was selected by the Levenberg-Marquardt algorithm, which showed less prediction error than other training algorithms.

5.3 Application of nanorobots for drug delivery

The development of micro and nano-electromechanical systems has provided the possibility of fabricating implantable robots for performing a variety of tasks, including the controlled delivery of drugs or genes. Because of the remarkable advances in nanotechnology, increasing interest has been attracted towards the development of nanorobots that are integrated with internal or external power supply, sensors, and AI. These smart structures are capable of information processing, signaling, sensing, actuation, communication, performing biological tasks at cellular levels, and localized delivery of drugs leading to the improved efficiency and reduced side effects of conventional therapeutics.

Nanorobots hold great promise for the detection of toxic agents and theranostic applications. Bionanorobot rule structure includes the navigation rules, collision avoidance, target identification rule, detection and attachment rule, drug delivery rule, mission complete rule, and activation of flush-out mode leading to the excretion of bio-nano robots. In molecular manufacturing automation, the application of AI provides the possibility to control the behavior or motion of nanorobots. Using the simulation and modeling techniques, collaborative and autonomous behaviors of nanorobots or nanorobotic-based drug delivery systems have been effectively simulated. Following the intravenous injection, bio-nanorobots are released into the bloodstream, and their swarming and swimming behaviors are facilitated by bio-actuation mechanisms. Swimming microrobots for controlled delivery of drugs, transient microrobot system for targeted drug delivery using touch-or nano-communication frameworks, or wirelessly-controlled and deeply penetrable microrobots have been suggested as novel forms of controlled-release drug delivery systems for targeted therapy in a variety of disorders, particularly the chronic ones that would be of great value in personalized medicine.

Magnetic microrobots can be used for ocular drug delivery. Wireless positioning and manipulation of drug delivery into the eye is a promising approach for targeted therapy with minimal invasiveness. Meanwhile, several issues have remained challenging, including those related to the fabrication process, controlling interactions with complex biological environments, and biocompatibility. Appropriate path planning is of critical importance for precise targeting and controlled drug delivery. Besides simulation of the dynamic environments, including the obstacles with different sizes and shapes, simulated annealing or a variety of algorithms such as the heuristic search, path planner, or swarm intelligence-based algorithms have been applied for detection of collisions, path planning and optimizing, target finding, or solving the problems associated with pathfinding. The quorum sensing technique has been employed to improve path-finding efficiency.

Furthermore, a novel technique that has been inspired by the bacterial for aging technique has been represented for optimizing robot path planning and finding the shortest path towards the target. An area coverage approach based on the genetic algorithm has also been proposed, which is characterized by the combination of online and offline path planning for coping with environmental uncertainties and overcoming obstacles during drug delivery. Turning angles and lengths of paths should be assessed to find the shortest and collision-free path. This might optimize the energy consumption of robots consisting of microsensing, micro actuating, and micro control units, drug reservoirs, and energy sources for targeted drug delivery within certain periods. Under the guidance of microcontrollers, the microrobot moves towards the target, followed by drug release. Because of the reusability, robots are able to bring back other drug reservoirs to the target site. The entrapped drug is released from the nanorobot via manipulation of the physiological conditions. However, any unexpected alteration of pH or temperature may negatively affect the drug release profile. In this respect, designing the externally-controlled nanomachines might be more appropriate for controlled drug delivery. Magnetoelectric nanorobots are promising nanodevices for drug delivery. Locomotion of these nanocarriers is controlled by magnetic fields, and their cargos are released in a controlled and site-specific fashion. For increased drug loading, nanowires have been pretreated with polydopamine leading to drug adsorption onto the surface of the nanorobot. For increased drug loading, nanowires have been pretreated with polydopamine leading to drug adsorption onto the surface of the nanorobot. Magnetic resonance imaging (MRI)-based drug delivery systems containing MRI propulsion and tracking modules, controller, and drug-loaded nanocapsules enhance the efficiency of therapeutics agents and reduce their side effects. Application of the nanorobotic system guided by MRI enables real-time monitoring of nanocapsules by an active targeting mechanism.

Following surface modification, metallic nanoshells, quantum dots, gold nanoparticles, or CNTs have been used as carrier modules of MRI-guided nanorobots. Meanwhile, the application of the appropriate algorithms to control the scenario carriers against the environmental perturbations and providing a 3D navigation path for enhanced targeting accuracy is necessary. DNA nanorobots for biosensing, triggering apoptosis, or drug delivery, have been activated by external nucleic acids capable of interacting with their complementary counterparts on nanorobots.

The application of ANNs for prediction and optimizing the performance of nanorobots embedded with biosensors and transducers is a promising approach for the detection of tumor cells and targeted drug delivery that might be of critical significance in cancer therapy and reduce adverse drug reactions. Detection of β-catenin and E-cadherin by these nanorobots facilitates target identification and localized delivery of therapeutics.

Nanorobots may also be applied for the controlled delivery of genes and overcoming the challenging issues associated with non-specific gene delivery methods. Moreover, nanorobots provide longer residence time for anti-cancer agents. Controlled drug delivery and the capability of nanorobots to carry drug combinations may provide pharmacological synergism and reduced drug resistance that might be of great significance in treating various cancer types. For instance, a combination of cyclosporine and doxorubicin has been shown to eradicate both leukemia and lymphoma.

For traveling toward the cancer cells, nanorobots should face an unstructured and cluttered environment in the bloodstream. This necessitates the application of suitable controllers and sensors for finding the right trajectory, overcoming the obstacles, discrimination of tumor cells (via detection of any difference between the temperature or electromagnetic field of the healthy and tumor cells), and delivery of the appropriate amount of drug. Following the determination of the concentration of glycoprotein molecules on the surface of cancer cells, cancer types can be identified by nanorobots. For instance, increased levels of CA19-9 and CA125 biomarkers indicate the presence of lymphoma and leukemia, respectively. Meanwhile, both of these markers are expressed in the aforementioned cancer types.

In fuzzy logic decision-making system can be applied for navigation, overcoming obstacles, preventing collisions with other nanorobots, tumor diagnosis, recognizing the disease stage, handling the uncertainties and noise, or delivery of the appropriate drug dosage, sensitivity, and concentration of CA19-9 and CA125 biomarkers have been considered as determining variables for discrimination of tumor cells. Because of the uncertainties associated with marker concentrations, the application of Mamdani fuzzy logic with flexible structure has been suggested for tumor diagnosis. Mamdani's approach provides the possibility to incorporate the uncertainties into the rule-based system or model the uncertainties associated with the navigation of bio-nano robots or the drug delivery process.

The robot consists of microsensing, micro actuating, micro control units, and a drug reservoir for targeted drug delivery within certain periods of time. Under the guidance of microcontrollers, the microrobot moves towards the target, followed by drug release. Because of the reusability, a microrobot is able to bring back another drug reservoir to the target site by incorporating the uncertainties into the rule-based system or modeling the uncertainties associated with the navigation of bio-nano robots or the drug delivery process.

Reduced processing time and power consumption are other beneficial aspects of Mamdani fuzzy logic, which provide increased execution time for bio nanorobots. After tumor diagnosis, drug dosage for intracellular delivery should be determined. The application of the Takagi-Sugeno fuzzy model provides the possibilities of linear mappings and obtaining the effective dose for intracellular delivery.

Following attachment to the tumor cell surface and drug injection by nano cannula, the mission complete rule guides the nanorobot towards the excretory system. In recent years, increasing interest has been attracted towards the development of medical capsule robots, the micro-systems capable of autonomous operation within the body for theranostic applications, monitoring disease progression, and drug delivery. Meanwhile, the commercially available capsule robots do not execute the algorithms for optimized drug delivery, which may be due to the absence of an active position control real-time localization.

In this respect, integration of a holding mechanism inside the capsule or application of a three-axis Helmholtzcoil capsule capable of rotational movement, magnetic locomotion system, or reed switch has been proposed for targeted drug delivery. For rapid development of medical capsule robots and intelligent drug delivery in a targeted manner, drug delivery capsules have been designed based on the combination of multiple functionalities, an intelligent scheduler, and a coil-magnet-piston mechanism for controlled drug release. The magnetic force and drug release profile have been modeled, followed by experimental verification.

5.4 Target fishing

Identification of the molecular targets might be of critical significance in the process of drug design. Target fishing (TF), by which the targets, mechanisms of action, or side effects of therapeutics are predicted, plays an important role in modern drug discovery. In this context, algorithms of machine learning and cheminformatics tool kits provide a piece of deeper knowledge about the structures of complex compounds and designing novel drug candidates against complex diseases. TF, by exploring the mechanisms of action of small molecules, identifying their target proteins, and speeding up the development process, may significantly reduce experimental costs. In drug discovery, bridging the biological and chemical space might be quite important. 2 and 3D descriptors can be applied to predict the targets of ligand probes considering their similarities to the reference molecules. In this context, high-affinity binding of diethylstilbestrol to the estrogen receptors has been revealed.

TF, which is based on computational-genomics, and proteomics-based methods, is a promising approach for the assessment of drug polypharmacology and molecular similarities. Using a large-scale TF approach based on the similarity rankings with data fusion, drug-relevant targets and potential toxicities have been predicted, indicating the significance of ligand-based TF in drug discovery. Furthermore, a search for the similarity of bioactivity profiles has been performed to the identification of the targets for uncharacterized compounds, suggesting novel targets for old therapeutics and prediction of the polypharmacological profiles of various compounds, adverse effects, or novel therapeutic indications. Considering the similarities between the ligands, the relationships between loperamide, methadone, and emetine with neurokinin, muscarinic, and adrenergic receptors (NK2, M3, α2, respectively) have been successfully characterized. Using the similarity search methods, the inhibitors of DNA methyltransferase and antithrombotic activity of the anti-diabetic drug glibenclamide have been identified. Furthermore, side-effect similarities and network analysis have enabled the identification of novel drug targets.

The application of phenotypic side-effect similarities followed by in vitro binding assay is a promising approach for characterizing unexpected relationships between drugs. Chemoproteomic technologies have provided the possibilities to investigate the mechanisms of action of a variety of drugs or bioactive small molecules and characterize drug-induced alterations in protein expression. Integrating the platforms of chemical proteomics into the initial stages of the process of drug discovery facilitates the identification of novel target proteins. Chemoproteomic fishing has enabled the identification of the modulators of brain glycogen phosphorylase, which regulates the metabolism of glucose.

Chemoproteomics has also been applied to characterize the properties of calixarene derivatives and their interactions with identified biomolecular targets, and targets of bioactive small molecules have been revealed that bioactive compounds exert their pharmacological effects via modulation of various targets, which could be unrelated structure, function, or sequence. In the cellular environment, the application of photoaffinity probes based on the carbine precursor, diazirine, has facilitated the identification of target proteins and interactome mapping.

For rationalizing the cytotoxic effects of aryl-aminopyridine derivatives against various cancer cell lines, screening compound libraries against targets has been performed considering the best correlation between in vitro cytotoxicity and docking scores. Based on the docking results, the modes of action of aminopyridine derivative simplicate disturbance of the cell cycle and signaling pathways via inhibition of various kinases. Furthermore, non-specific inhibition of tyrosine and cyclin-dependent kinases has resulted in cytotoxic effects. These types of findings can be utilized for the modification of compounds and the development of drugs capable of targeting the protein implicated in the survival and proliferation of cancer cells.

TF using the cross-docking approach can be performed for the identification of novel protein-drug interactions. This might be useful for explaining various types of side effects or suggesting new modes of action. For instance, peroxisome proliferator-activated receptor-γ has been predicted as a target of ethacrynic acid that may justify the hyperglycemia induced by this diuretic. The novel repositioning opportunities of drugs or potential mechanisms of adverse reactions can be predicted by cross-docking.

For investigating the effects and mechanisms of action of natural products in the treatment of atherosclerosis, sepsis, or migraine, TF has been performed to identify the candidate targets and target compound interactions. Capsaicin has shown therapeutic potential against a variety of disorders. In order to better understand the mechanisms of action of this alkaloid, its potential targets have been predicted by Pharm Mapper, followed by confirmation via molecular docking and chemical protein interactome. Based on the findings, capsaicin is a potent inhibitor of the isoenzymes of carbonic anhydrase. A pharmacophore-based TF approach has been employed to predict the targets of isoquinoline alkaloids with protective effects against inflammation, pain, infections, or cancer. TF approaches have also been applied to predict the potential targets and molecular mechanisms of the flavonoid baicalein. It was shown that baicalein remarkably reduces the generation of intracellular nitric oxide and reactive oxygen species and exhibits protective effects against the neurotoxicity induced by N-methyl-D-aspartic acid receptors indicating the antiparkinsonian effect of this flavonoid.

Furthermore, chemical proteomics strategies can be used for the identification of the binding partners of natural products, including antibacterial and cytotoxic agents. For target identification of the electrophilic natural products, activity-based protein profiling (ABPP) is a promising approach. Competitive ABPP has been applied for the development of the inhibitors of serine hydrolase with therapeutic potential against a variety of disorders.

Meanwhile, the indirect nature of most of the identification approaches and the non-specific binding of some proteins are challenging issues in chemical proteomics that necessitate the application of advanced quantitative proteomics techniques and suitable linkers. Regarding the special types of diseases in which conventional drugs could be associated with serious side effects, the identification of new macromolecular targets may provide therapeutics with increased activities and reduced side effects. Molecular modeling has enabled the identification of potential targets for novel anti-leishmanial agents. Following the TF study, 4-phenyl-1 and 3-thiazol-2-amines have been represented as suitable scaffolds for designing selective antileishmanial drugs with improved activities. TF tools have also proved to be useful for predicting targets for anti-tuberculosis drugs. DNA gyrase and RNA polymerase have been successfully predicted as targets of the antibacterial agent CBR-2092.

In difficult-to-treat diseases such as Chagas disease, in which the currently available drugs are associated with numerous side effects and low efficiency, identifying novel molecular targets and developing of their inhibitors provide improved therapeutic outcomes. The effects and mechanism of action of the antidepressant sertraline against the various strains of Trypanosomacruzi have been investigated by TF. The chemogenomics strategy was used to identify several similar targets in the parasite. Based on the findings, sertraline with multi-target characteristics affects the bioenergetic metabolism of Trypanosoma cruzi. In general, TF methods are based on screening procedures, including machine learning algorithms, selection of the reference ligands, and determining the appropriateness of targets. For target ranking or prioritization, various TF methods, including those based on the ranking perceptrons algorithms and support vector machines, have been applied. Using a network-based inference method, montelukast has been identified as the inhibitor of dipeptidyl-peptidase-4. Furthermore, polypharmacological profiles of ketoconazole, diclofenac, itraconazole, and simvastatin on the estrogen receptors have been evaluated.

Based on the necessity of validating the prediction and classification methods, machine learning methods have been used for cross-validation. Retrospective analysis can also be used for the validation of some TF methods. Ligand-centric and target-centric methods can be used to predict the activity of test ligands against the corresponding targets.

Target-centric methods are usually based on multi-target QSAR models or unsupervised learning approaches, and numerous targets have been considered by ligand-centric methods.

In a study conducted by Peón et al., the methods of ligand-centric target predictions have been systematically validated using various clinically-used drugs, and novel estimates regarding the polypharmacological profiles of drugs have been obtained.

Meanwhile, an experimental confirmation appears more appropriate for the validation of the predictive methods. Over the last decade, parallel screening has been suggested as a promising approach for rational TF and pharmacological profiling of the chemicals. ANN-based methods minimize the number of experiments and costs, optimize drug release profiles, or estimate pharmacodynamic and pharmacokinetic profiles of drugs. In cancer therapy, the application of a fuzzy logic-based intelligent system is useful for diagnostic applications, improved drug delivery efficiency and navigation of bio-nano robots, and reduced false-positive rates.

5.5 Drug safety

• Introduction

Drug safety is a major challenge while bringing new drugs to market. Unexpected toxicities are a major source of attrition during clinical trials, and post-marketing safety concerns cause unnecessary morbidity and mortality. Adverse events (AEs), or adverse drug reactions (ADRs) when causality is demonstrated, are unexpected effects occurring from a normal dosage of the drug. The economic, social, and health burden of toxicity and safety assessment is an essential and pressing public health concern. Before a drug is approved, clinical trials ensure that this drug is safe and effective for its intended use. Once a drug is marketed, drugs are monitored through AE reports ensuring that a drug's safety information is up to date, a process called pharmacovigilance (PV). However, neither of these processes are error proof as clinical trials suffer from structural limitations. For example, it is impossible to test for all potential synergistic effects or to conduct trials on populations large enough to detect rare AEs.

Until recently, women and the elderly were considered special sub-groups for clinical trials. These trials have focused on designing drugs for the average patient even at a time when there are increasing calls for precision medicine to enable the "right drug at the right dose to the right patient".Once drugs are approved, it is the purview of programs to monitor drug safety. These agencies use databases of spontaneously collected AE reports to flag leads and perform confirmatory follow-up analyses. However, these spontaneous reports are known to suffer from biases such as under-reporting, which is especially troublesome for rare events and drug-drug interactions (DDIs). The research community has turned to statistical and computational approaches to address these limitations and supplement its PV toolbox.

Over the past decade, we have seen two phenomena occur:

(1) The explosion of freely accessible databases of medical, chemical, and pharmacological knowledge, along with the rapid adoption of electronic health record (EHR) systems, stimulated by the Health Information Technology for Economic and Clinical Health (HITECH) Act iii.

(2) The development of novel computational methods in the realm of machine learning (ML) and deep learning (DL) is a popular re-branding of neural networks –catalyzed by the exponential increase in computing power and data availability.

- **Pre-clinical Drug Safety**

AI techniques have shown to play an important role in pre-market drug safety, especially in the area of toxicity evaluation. Drug toxicity determination is the main step in drug design and involves identifying the AEs of chemicals on humans, plants, animals, and the environment.

Pre-clinical evaluations are a necessity for preventing toxic drugs from reaching clinical trials. Despite this, high toxicity is still a major contributor to drug failure accounting for two-thirds of post-market drug withdrawals and for one-fifth of failures during clinical trials. Thus, accurate toxicity estimates are necessary for ensuring drug safety and can help reduce the cost and development time of bringing new drugs to market. Animal studies have historically been the most conventional approach taken to assess toxicity. However, these studies are constrained by cost, time, and ethical considerations. Numerous computational in silicon approaches have demonstrated utility in estimating the toxicity of drug candidates. These approaches predict toxicity by evaluating various features of the drug and include target-based predictions and Quantitative Structure-Activity Relationships (QSAR).

• ML methods:

Features of QSAR are summarized in Table 3, and the associated ML methods are discussed in Table4. Other applied branches of AI like DL and CNN are discussed later in this section.

CLASSIFICATION METHODS	APPLICATIONS
Support vector machines	• **Prediction of the activity of enzyme inhibitors or rate-limited drug absorption** • **Example: In a QSAR study, 1,4-dihydropyridine calcium channel antagonists have been screened by least squares support vector machine**
Supervised learning algorithms	• **Prediction of drug-target interactions** • **Example: regularized least squares classifier for prediction of drug-target interactions** • **Remark: Semi-supervised link prediction classifier has shown high performance in predicting drug target interactions**
Combination of Gaussian interaction profile kernels and genomic and chemical kernels	• **Better predictivepower**

Table 19 Features of QSAR

TargeTox:

It leverages protein target data with a network-based approach and gradient boosting to identify potentially toxic drugs. This approach builds protein networks using a distance metric following the assumption that neighboring biological entities share functional roles, thus hypothesizing that toxicity responses can be isolated to specific network regions. The built networks, pharmacological, and functional impact data from the public datasets, like DrugBankxiand ChEMBL, comprise the model features.

A gradient boosting classifier is then applied to develop a quantitative toxicity prediction score for each drug. While the authors specifically discuss a gradient boosting ensemble approach, any classifier with a regularization function and the capacity to handle non-linear relationships can be applied. TargeTox has multiple model variants based on which distance metric is used for network calculation. The top-performing approach uses a diffusion state distance (DSD) with a subset of reference points to calculate the distance to the closest protein bound by a drug candidate. This method achieved an AUC of 743 with a sensitivity of 0.75 and specificity of 0.658 when trained and tested on data from Drug Bank and Clinical trials with 5-fold cross-validation. The novelty of TargeTox is its ability to generate protein network data as well as combine other pharmacological and functional features into an ML classifier for toxicity prediction.

PrOCTOR:

It is a target-based toxicity prediction software that, in addition to network information, also incorporates chemical properties into its scoring. To develop a PrOCTOR score, the algorithm combines chemical structure properties of the drug candidate (e.g.molecular weight, polar surface area, quantitative estimate of drug-likeness (QED)) along with protein target information (e.g., network connectivity, tissue-specific expression). Drug target data is extracted from public datasets, including DrugBank, GTExxiii, and ExACxiv. Compared toTargeTox, the PrOCTOR model includes many more features with a total of 48 variables (34 target-based, 10 structure, and 4 drug-likeness) per drug compound model. A random forest classifier is used on the 48-feature model to develop a PrOCTOR score which assesses the likelihood of toxicity. This model constructs 50 decision trees using a subset of the features and uses the tree consensus to predict the outcome. PrOCTOR showed high performance (AUC=0.83) and accuracy (ACC = 0.75) with high sensitivity (0.75) and specificity (0.74) when trained on a set of 784FDA drugs with 10-fold cross-validation. PrOCTOR's ability to leverage multiple types of target and structure-based features for toxicity prediction places set sits above many other target-based algorithms.

• **Deep learning methods:**

Furthermore, Deep learning methods are also employed in QSAR for pre-clinical drug safety procedures. DL is an extension of ANNs which uses a hierarchy of ANNs to learn useful features from raw data. A Merck-sponsored Kaggle competition in 2012 introduced DL to the field of drug discovery. The winning team used DL on a set of diverse QSAR data sets to predict activity values for various compounds. Recently, numerous studies of toxicity modeling have used DL approaches. To assess hepatotoxicity, Xu et al. used DL to build drug-induced liver injury (DILI) prediction models with chemical structure data. The authors used a recurrent neural network to construct the models. The best model was trained on 475 drugs and predicted an external validation set of about 200 drugs with an accuracy of 86.9%, sensitivity of 82.5%, and specificity of 92.9%. This model outperformed previously reported DILI prediction models.

• **Deep convolutional neural networks (CNNs)**

They are a class of DL networks that learn representations of raw images from pixel information as a hierarchy of images from which features can be extracted and used to classify complex patterns. CNN's have been used to predict toxicity from images of cells pre-treated with a set of drugs. This approach effectively predicted a broad spectrum of toxicity mechanisms from different drugs, nuclear stains, and cell lines. Tong et al. also used a CNN strategy in a protein structure analysis task. Specifically, a 3D CNN approach was used to analyze amino acid microenvironments and predict the effects of mutations on protein structure. No prior knowledge or feature assumptions were required for this prediction task.

And the approach demonstrated a two-fold increase in accuracy prediction compared with models that require hand-selected features. Other DL approaches that have been used to assess drug toxicity include autoencoders, generative adversarial networks (GANs), and long-short-term memory, among others.

• Post-marketingsurveillance

In 1962, it was revealed that thousands of babies were born with malformed limbs because thalidomide, a mild sleeping pill, had no contraindications for pregnant women to whom it was often prescribed off-label. The WHO "Programme for International Drug Monitoring" xv was created following this disaster. Since 1978, the Uppsala Monitoring Centre (UMC) in Sweden is the global coordinator for PV in collaboration with the WHO and counts 134 full member countries with national agencies supporting patient safety and drug AE reporting systems. These initiatives are proof that safety assessment in clinical trials has its limit and that drug safety needs to be actively monitored during the entire market life of drugs.

The classical methods to evaluate causality include the Naranjo algorithm, the Venulet algorithm, and the World Health Organization- Upsala Monitoring Centre (WHO-UMC) system for standardized case causality assessment, among others. But with known shortcomings, such as confounding biases and under-reporting, the attention has shifted to other data sources and advanced computational methods that could replace or complement existing resources. Below we discuss the approaches and data sources that can support post-marketing PV along with the associated AI-driven methods needed to extract information and learn from it.

SystemPharmacology

System pharmacology is the study of drug action using principles from systems biology, considering the effect of the drug on the entire system rather than a single target or metabolizing enzyme. This approach promises to explain unexpected drug effects that may result from complex interactions of targets and pathways. The application of systems pharmacology to adverse drug events differs from its use in drug discovery in that it's focused on off-target effects and clinical observations of adverse reactions. In addition, it is one of the most data-rich approaches to drug safety for in silico ADR mining. As a consequence of the rich data sources available, investigators in system pharmacology for adverse drug effects (ADEs) now have methods of choice involving network approaches and the ability to integrate multiple types of features. Lorberbaum et al. proposed the modular assembly of drug safety subnetworks (MADSS), where they generated protein networks using knowledge bases that were pruned with literature mining, genome-wide association study (GWAS) data, assigned phenotype target with DrugBank and ChEMBL, and finally, trained random forest models on network metrics to predict new drugs causing AEs. Raja et al. focused on DDIs by mining the literature to integrate drug-gene interactions (DGIs) at different scales and trained random forest models to predict DDIs with a gold standard corpus, focusing specifically on cutaneous diseases. Sornalakshmi et al. trained SVM models on similarity measures such as 2D molecular structure similarity, 3D pharmacologic similarity, interaction profile fingerprint

(IPF) similarity, target similarity, and ADE similarity from DrugBank and SIDERxvito predict drug pairs likely to interact with each other based on a literature-based gold standard. Xu et al. used various pharmaceutical compound datasets and neural networks to encode these drugs using the undirected graph recursive neural networks (UG-RNN) introduced by Luscietal. And classified them between DILI positive and DILI negative compounds. Herrero et al. used pharmacokinetic(PK) and pharmacodynamic(PD) properties from DrugBank and other sources, along with drug-enzymes relationship data, to build neural networks supervised models taking Lexicompxvii and Vidal compendia xviii as ground truth for DDI labels. All of the above approaches heavily rely on molecular features directly linked to these drugs along with phenotypic evidence of their effects, and the source datasets are usually open. However, the clinical information used is often limited to specific outcomes, missing the longitudinal patient medical history and all the other clinical covariates. In contrast, EHRs are closed datasets that have been used to compensate for the episodic aspect of SRS and provide observational data captured during medical encounters.

EHR mining

Stimulated by the HITECH Act, the rapid and widespread adoption of EHRs that we have witnessed this past decade has also enabled researchers to tap into these rich and noisy sources of clinical data for PV. EHR data stand out in their challenging heterogeneity: these temporal data sources include categorical data such as diagnostic, procedure, and medication codes, but also continuous laboratory tests and measurement values, along with large volumes of semi-structured and unstructured medical notes and reports.

Structured EHR data

Structured data such as diagnoses, procedures, medications, and laboratory tests present the advantage of requiring the least pre-processing for ML approaches. Zhao et al. studied nine different weighting strategies regarding how to use drugs, diagnoses, and measurements as features in supervised learning algorithms for ADR prediction.

Bayesian methods

They have been popular in modeling medical outcomes. Benefiting from a knowledge-rich domain, a variety of Bayesian approaches have been used for adverse event prediction by including prior medical knowledge. Bekker et al. used Bayesian network representations to model the effect of drugs on the progression of multiple co-morbidities using prescriptions and diagnoses from primary care data. Moghaddass et al. proposed to generalize the self-controlled case series (SCCS) with a multivariate hierarchical Bayesian model to leverage latent factor analysis (LFA) and bring more interpretability regarding the effects of transient multi-drug exposures on a collection of health outcomes. As an alternative, Morel et al. proposed another multivariate SCCS method based on the convolution of step functions with point drug exposures to estimate the effect of longitudinal features. Kuang et al. directly followed up with that multiple SCCS and presented a baseline regularization to take into account the individual-specific, time-dependent occurrence rate of AEs. More recently, they have also presented a version of that model for drug repurposing. Rather than predicting discrete outcomes, it is also possible to model drug responses by predicting dynamic time series of observational data to select the best treatment courses. Xu et al. estimated the individualized treatment response (ITR) curve with Bayesian non-parametric (BNP). They modeled creatinine time series response of treatments used in managing kidney function and demonstrated a gain in accuracy compared to baseline models. Structured data have the advantage of being easily pre-processed for ML and DL algorithms, but they also have to rely on mappings, data structures, and terminologies that could impede reproducibility.

Beyond structured data, which presents both standardization and mapping challenges and may not be readily accessible, biomedical and clinical corpora represent a valuable resource. More importantly, because they are primarily designed for billing purposes, EHR databases present a number of biases, including confounding bias and selection bias, and do not provide the whole picture of their patient's care trajectory.

Natural Language Processing (NLP)

These methods are essential in this area to extract concepts and apply ML or learn embedding representations of these documents to make predictions directly. Abacha et al. developed a hybrid feature-based and kernel-based system for DDI detection and classification applied to the DDI-Extraction-2013 corpus. That corpus contained 1017 medical texts, including abstracts from MEDLINE and documents describing DDIs from the DrugBank database, annotated with DDIs and pharmacological substances for the supervision of the learning task. Mower et al. built the embedding of semantic predications (ESP) by extracting concept-relationship-concept triples from the literature with the SemRepNLP systems xix. They trained a kNN model with the Exploring and Understanding ADRs by Integrative Mining of Clinical Records and Biomedical Knowledge (EU-ADR) and the Observational Medical Outcomes Partnership (OMOP) datasets, two national networks that have defined common data models as ground truth and showed good generalization performances to predict binary ADE outcomes. Kim et al. opted for a naïve Bayes classifier to predict the likelihood of ADR in textual data from expert opinion on ADR case reports from the Korean Adverse Event Reporting System database. NLP has dramatically benefited from advances in DL in recent years to build better language models, with the development of word embeddings, sequence-to-sequence (seq2seq) learning, and, more recently, attention mechanisms. The clinical domain has always been a challenging field of application for NLP, and these novel methods have been promptly applied to PV problems.

Language models can be trained using the biomedical literature and then applied to clinical notes, as demonstrated by Dev et al., where the authors used MEDLINE to learn a better representation of concepts found in narrative logs for the classification of ADEs. A recurrent theme in NLP for the detection of the drug to AE relationship prediction is the need first to detect the concept (i.e., Named Entity Recognition (NER)) and then perform the learning task. These two tasks, as shown in the studies previously mentioned, can both be conducted with neural networks. With its natural properties of connections and weights, DL enables multi-task learning (MTL), an approach that consists of sharing the weights of the neural networks between multiple tasks to improve overall performance. Zhang et al. used this technique to jointly learn NER in texts for AE cases and ADE classification between serious and non-serious effects. Similarly, Li et al. applied bi LSTM networks to the Medication, Indication, and Adverse Drug Events (MADE) 1.0 challenge for NER with a conditional random field network and for relations extraction with an attention mechanism. More recently and using the same dataset, Yang et al. developed a similar LSTM model for NER but extracted relations between concepts and ADEs by comparing SVM and random forests. These NLP techniques have also been used with data collected on social media and in online health communities. There is evidence that users on social media disseminate information comparable to ICSRs, and ADEs can be classified from these high-noise data sources. Post-marketing PV has been conducted using Twitter data with embedding techniques and bi LSTM deep classifiers that outperform conditional random field methods, discussion forums, or more domain-specific health social networking sites.

5.6 Antimicrobial resistance

• Introduction

The modern era of antibiotics began with a fortuitous discovery by Fleming in 1928. (102) Since then, antibiotics have saved many patients with infections, including dental infections. However, the wide clinical application of antibiotics has not only led to the emergence of drug resistance but also introduced the threat of super-resistant bacteria. It is estimated that antimicrobial resistance (AMR) will cause approximately 10 million deaths every year, and the economic cost of AMR is expected to exceed $100 billion by 2050. Thus, coordinated efforts to implement new policies and renew research efforts to manage the AMR crisis are urgently needed. For example, the U.S. Food and Drug Administration (FDA) has offered provisions to stipulate the types, quantities, and frequencies of antibiotic use. In 2006, the European Union proposed a total ban on adding antibiotics to livestock feed.

In China, the National Action Plan to Contain Antimicrobial Resistance was published in 2016. Although people have paid more attention to AMR, the overall situation is deteriorating, and we still need to develop antimicrobial peptides (AMPs), antibiotic combinations, and monitoring systems to effectively control AMR. In recent years, artificial intelligence has shown significant performance in AMR control. For example, sequencing-based AI applications have been employed to study AMR. In addition, collecting clinical data to build clinical decision support systems could help physicians monitor trends in AMR to increase the rational use of antibiotics. Furthermore, AI applications are widely used for designing new antibiotics and synergistic drug combination investigations. However, since most of the previous reviews about AMR have been made from a structural and molecular mechanism perspective, this study aims to offer a systematic review for AI-based applications in AMR control from different angles of a predictive AMR model, antibiotic-resistant infections, rational use of antibiotics, AMPs and antibiotic combinations.

? Commonly used artificial intelligence algorithms for AMR
The most widely used artificial intelligence algorithms for AMR include naïve Bayes (NB), decision trees (DT), random forests (RF), support vector machines (SVM), and artificial neural networks (ANN).

? Naïve Bayes
Naïve Bayes is a classification method based on Bayes' theorem with independent assumptions of each feature. For a given training dataset, the input/output joint probability distribution is calculated. Recent studies have typically employed the naïve Bayes model to monitor AMR. For example, Rezaei-Hachesu et al. used naïve Bayes and a priori algorithms to determine the key factor of resistance and to extract resistant patterns. In addition, Choisyetal used naïve Bayes to estimate the probabilities of ineffective treatment due to AMR.

- **Decision tree**

The decision tree is usually used for classification. The learning process of a decision tree usually consists of three steps:

(1) Feature selection
(2) Decision tree generation
(3) Decision tree pruning

The primary foundation of these steps mostly originates from ID3, C4.5, and CART. The decision tree model is often used to allocate medical resources appropriately by estimating the burden of AMR. For example, Reynolds et al. employed a decision tree model to estimate healthcare utilization and cost for AMR, demonstrating that the reduction in AMR or improvement of antibiotic selection could lead to substantial savings. Voermans et al. used a procalcitonin (PCT)-based decision tree model to guide antibiotic use, which resulted in shorter treatment duration and lower total dosages.

- **Random forest**

Random forest is an ensemble algorithm that employs multiple decision trees to improve accuracy and reliability. It uses two key concepts. One is a random sampling from the training set, which means that some samples will be used multiple times in a tree. The other is a random subset of features, meaning that the performance of a single tree in a random forest may be reduced, but as the number of trees increases, the random forest usually converges to a lower generalization error. Random forest models have been commonly used to predict antibiotic combinations. For example, Chandrasekaran et al. employed a random forest model to predict effective antibiotic combination therapies using chemogenomics data and orthology, which has a simple and regular structure, low computing complexity (n2/2), and high generalization performance (AUC for synergy = 0.79). However, since chemogenomics data are inadequate, Mason et al. employed the molecular fingerprint as a feature to improve the predictive power of the aforementioned models.

• **Support vector machine**

A support vector machine (SVM) is a binary classification model that identifies a partitioning hyperplane in the sample space to separate samples into different classes. Recent studies have often employed SVM models to predict AMR phenol types, i.e., 'resistant' or 'susceptible'. For example, Her et al. predicted whether E.coli are resistant to antibiotics using SVM models. Results demonstrated that this model achieved average accurate predictions up to 0.95 (based on the AUC). In addition, Liu et al. employed SVM models to examine the resistance of five drugs (tetracycline, ampicillin, sulfisoxazole, trimethoprim, and enrofloxacin), the results of which showed that the accuracy of the model achieves 90% or greater. Therefore, we consider SVM models as potential tools for AMR surveillance and clinical diagnosis.

• **Artificial neural network**

Artificial neural networks are abstract mathematical models that use loosely modeled neurons in the human brain to transmit information through weighted, interconnected computer units or "neuron" layers.

The training algorithm for neural networks is to minimize the activation function of weights ωi and biases b. Recently, Stokes et al. identified new antibiotics without any prior assumptions using a deep learning approach, one of the artificial neural networks. Next, we will use a deep learning approach to design new antibiotics and optimize existing molecules, which could mark a paradigm shift for future antibiotic discovery.

- **Applications of artificial intelligence for antimicrobial resistance (AMR)**

Antibiotics are small molecules that can inhibit or kill bacteria and are often used to treat bacterial infections in clinics. Unfortunately, the abuse of antibiotics results in AMR. As AMR significantly decreases antibiotic therapeutic efficacy, it is vital for us to track its emergence and spread. Currently, two typical methods are widely used to diagnose AMR. One is antimicrobial susceptibility testing (AST), and the other is whole-genome sequencing for antimicrobial susceptibility testing (WGSAST). AST is the classic method to quantify antimicrobial resistance levels, but it is neither efficient nor does it explain the mechanism of AMR.

WGS-AST provides rapid, consistent, and accurate diagnosis for AMR, but it requires large and high-dimensional datasets to extract information effectively. Thus, artificial intelligence technologies are employed to improve upon previous methods as follows. To improve AST methods, Inglis et al. used a combined method of flow cytometer antimicrobial susceptibility testing (FAST) and supervised machine learning to perform antimicrobial susceptibility testing. This type of AI method generates a reliable result in less than 3 h. Moreover, Lechowicz et al. reduced the amount of time to perform AST from 24 h to 30 min by developing an IR-spectrometer method that combines infrared (IR) spectroscopy with artificial neural network.

CHAPTER SIX

OPERATIVE DENTISTRY

"Artificial Intelligence, deep learning, machine learning — whatever you're doing if you don't understand it — learn it. Because otherwise you're going to be a dinosaur within 3 years."
Mark Cuban

Periapical granulomas, abscesses, and cysts are the most common periapical lesions that are evident on radiographs, but some may go unnoticed as images may be noisy or have low contrast. AI can accurately locate tooth areas prone to caries and complex periapical pathoses, define the boundaries of lesions in a more precise way and enable their differentiation. Detection and characterization of proximal caries is possible with the help of Logic on Caries Detector.(103,104) AI can help in analyzing the lifespan of different restorative materials and to choose them wisely for suitable cases(105) and aid in successfully locating the minor apical foramen (AF) thereby strengthening the accuracy of working length.(106)

In a study conducted by Orhan et al.(66), using method of DCNN, CBCT images of periapical pathosis were assessed with 92.8% reliability. In another study conducted by Rhienmora et al. (107) virtual reality (VR) and an augmented reality (AR) dental training simulator utilizing a haptic device were developed. The simulators utilize volumetric force feedback computation and real time modification of the volumetric data. They include a virtual mirror to facilitate indirect vision during a simulated operation. The AR environment allows students to practice surgery in correct postures by combining the 3D tooth and tool models with the real world view and displaying the result through a video see-through head-mounted display (HMD). Preliminary results from an initial evaluation show that the system is a promising tool to supplement dental training and that there are advantages of the AR over the VR approach.

In a study by Bhatia A. et al. (108), using Bayesian network, decision making tool of dental caries was designed. It consists of caries, cavity, fistula, swelling, food lodgment, previous broken filing, sensitivity, pain, pain on percussion, partial denture, pulp exposure, high filing as sign-symptom nodes and palliative, RCT, Relieve high points, direct pulp capping, indirect pulp capping, resolution as treatment nodes. This could help to treat the endodontic patient with high level of confidence and hence improve the overall performance.This research is constrained to dental caries only, but can incorporate other oral diseases. AL bahbah AA et al. (109), presented tooth caries identification system based on SVM trained by using practical swarm optimization (PSO). The proposed approach utilizes inter-pixel auto correlation as input features. Experimental results prove that the proposed approach can detect tooth caries efficiently. Furthermore, it is clear that the classification accuracy is very good. In addition, the proposed approach of tooth caries detection outperforms the diagnosing process performed by a rule-based computer assisted program and a group of dentists.

With the minute margins of error in endodontic surgery, training in manual dexterity and proper instrument handling are crucial components. Important parameters include tool path, tool angulation, and force applied. Too great a force can cause overdrilling or in extreme cases perforation of the tooth. Too small a force can cause thermal irritation possibly resulting in tissue necrosis. Despite the importance of correct use of force, this is the dimension on which students receive the least tutorial feedback since force information is typically not available in traditional training settings. Su Yin M. et al. (110), used Haptic feedback to train correct application of force in Endodontic Surgery. Feedback is conveyed to the student graphically and the correct amount of force to apply is trained haptically. The simulator is rewound and the student is asked to redo the stage where the error occurred. Preliminary evaluation against a control group of students who received only feedback concerning outcome shows the feedback mechanism to be effective.

CHAPTER SEVEN

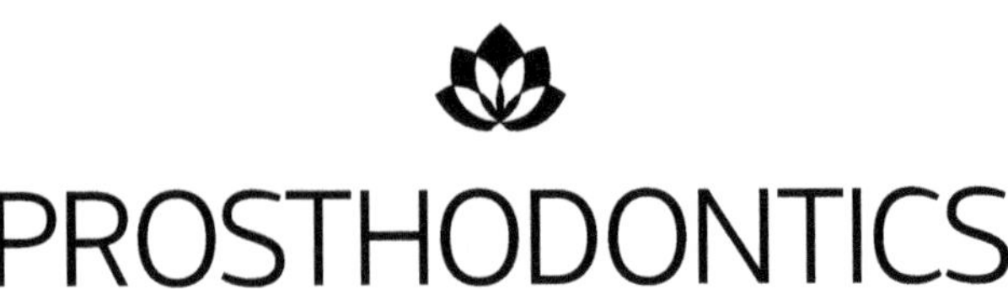

PROSTHODONTICS

"The techniques of artificial intelligence are to the mind what bureaucracy is to human social interaction."

Terry Winograd

When it comes down to implementing ANN in clinical practice, it has sufficient precision for the design and chairside manufacturing of dental prostheses, based on digital image acquisition following tooth cusps assessment.(103) It can have a great potential in investigating the properties of dental materials such as chemical stability, wear resistance, and flexural strength.(104) AI along with some designing software also aid the dentist to design the best possible and aesthetic prosthesis for patients while considering a number of variables like anthropological calculations, facial measurements, ethnicity and even patient's desire.(111)(112)

The fabrication of the prosthesis is currently carried out with CAD-CAM technologies like subtractive milling and additive manufacturing technologies like 3D printing. It has replaced the time consuming and laborious process of conventional casting and simultaneously drastically reduced the human errors in the final prosthesis. These technologies can also be used to fabricate accurate orthodontic plates and appliances too.(113) AI combined with designing software's can aid the dentist to design the best possible and aesthetic prostheses considering number of factors like facial measurements, anthropological calculations, ethnicity and patient desire. AI plays a major role in identifying the type of bone, cortical thickness for making precise surgical guides for placing implants. The time consuming and laborious process of conventional casting is replaced by the use of CAD-CAM technology(113) which creates a 2D and 3D models thereby reducing human errors. Virtual reality simulation (VRS) technology can be used to simulate the facial profiles post treatment. This enables the dentist to efficiently design the esthetics and also acts as a motivational tool for the patient(28).

Deniz ST et al. (114), compared the performance of artificial neural network (ANN) model with the results of in vitro experiments. For these experiments, maxillary molars of four different denture teeth were subjected to tea, coffee, cola, cherry juice, distilled water. Vickers microhardness and surface roughness values were measured. Subsequently, ANN model for the prediction of microhardness and surface roughness of different denture teeth were examined. A back-propagation ANN has been used to develop a model relating to the amount of microhardness and surface roughness. The independent variables of the model are distilled water, tea, filtered coffee, cola, cherry juice, time and denture teeth. Microhardness and surfaceroughness were chosen as the dependent variables. According to the results, a neural network architecture having one input layer with ten neurons, two hidden layers with six neurons, one output layer with two neurons and anepochsizeof 48 gives better prediction.

Matching the color of a natural tooth with a ceramic restoration is still one of the most challenging topics in esthetic prosthodontics. Li H. et al. (115), used GA+BP Neural Network based computer color matching predictor to reduce the influence of subjective factors by technicians in their study. Utilization of genetic algorithm (GA) to optimize the initial weights and threshold values in BPNN improves the precision and prediction robustness of the color matching in restorative dentistry.

Mine Y. et al.(116), compared two machine learning algorithms, ANN-based deep learning and the random forest algorithm, to determine the compounding amount of pigmentation in maxillofacial prosthesis. They used 52 silicone elastomer specimens of varying colors and measured the CIE 1976 L* a*b* color space information using a spectro photometer on the input dataset. The output of these algorithms indicated the compounding amount of four pigments. They determined the color differences between the real skin color of five research participants (22.3 ± 1.7 years) and that of the silicone elastomer specimens fabricated based on the algorithm predictions using the CIEDE00 ΔE00 color system. The color differences (ΔE00 value) between the real skin color and silicone elastomer validation specimens were 3.45 ± 0.87 (ANN) and 5.54 ± 1.41 (random forest), which indicates that the deep ANN approach produced superior results with respect to the ΔE00 value compared with the random forest algorithm.

Chen Q. et al.(117) , developed an ontological paradigm to developing a clinical decision support model for specific design of removable partial dentures (RPDs). During the case-based reasoning process, a cosine similarity algorithm was applied to calculate similarity values between input patients and standard ontology cases. A group of designs from the most similar cases were output as the final results.To evaluate this model, the output designs of RPDs for 104 randomly selected patients were compared with those selected by professionals. An area under the curve of the receiver operating characteristic (AUC-ROC) was created by plotting true-positive rates against the false-positive rate at various threshold settings. The precision at position 5 of the retrieved cases was 0.67 and at the top of the curve it was 0.96, both of which are very high. The mean average of precision (MAP) was 0.61 and the normalized discounted cumulative gain (NDCG) was 0.74 both of which confirmed the efficient performance of our model. All the metrics demonstrated the efficiency of this model.

CHAPTER EIGHT

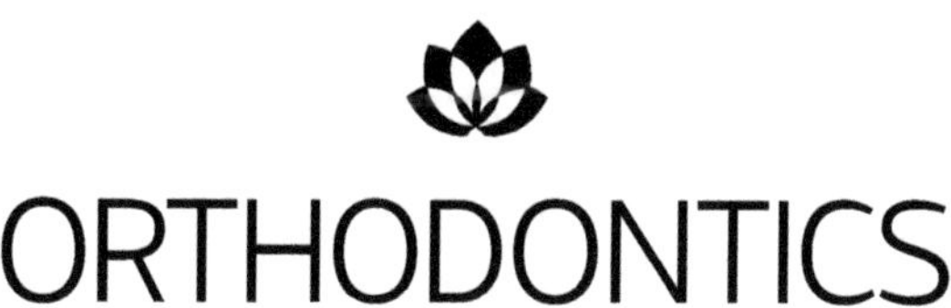

ORTHODONTICS

"Artificial Intelligence is the new electricity."
Andrew Ng

In orthodontics, diagnosis forms the crux of the treatment. When a proposed model was trained in this aspect to assess the cranio facial skeletal and dental abnormalities in cephalometry followed by comparison with an expert opinion, the agreement between them was found to be equivalent. In addition,the model pointed out contradictions presented in the data that were not noticed by the orthodontists, thereby highlighting the contribution of AI in orthodontic decision support.(118) It can also be used to provide orthodontic consultations to general practitioners for the alignment of crowded lower teeth.(119) Further progressing to the role of AI in treatment planning, the neural networks when optimally trained with respect to lower third molars are found to have high specificity and sensitivity equivalent to specialist consultation in categorizing tooth to "gold standard" based on NIH consensus criteria.(120)

GAs and ANN are a promising tool for predicting the sizes of unerupted canines and premolars with greater accuracy in the mixed dentition period(5) and can also be optimized for predicting the tooth surface loss which is a universal problem that involves an irreversible, multifactorial, non-carious, physiologic, pathologic,or functional loss of dental hard tissues.(121)

Added to this, the ANN can be employed to determine if extractions are necessary before orthodontic treatment,(106) in predicting tooth movements and final outcome of the treatment(122) , to predict orthodontic treatment plans, anchorage patterns(123), to identify the factors that influence decision-making before orthodontic treatment. Customized aligner-based orthodontics can improve case acceptance when combined with latest technologies. In the field of orthodontics the software can perform a number of analysis on radiographs and photographs that aid in diagnosis and treatment planning.(124)(125)

With the advent of intra-oral scanners and cameras the ordeal of making a dental impression is also disappearing soon and is being replaced by digital impressions(126) and the above data is fed into the system; These digital impressions are not only quicker and more accurate but also eliminate all the laboratory steps thus drastically reducing the number of errors. With the help of Artificial Intelligence, the computer can actually guide the dentist during the entire procedure of making a digital impression and aid in making an ideal impression. (127) Based on the information that is fed into the system, the set algorithms and statistical analysis, the AI software helps to predict tooth movement and final outcome of treatment too.

CHAPTER NINE

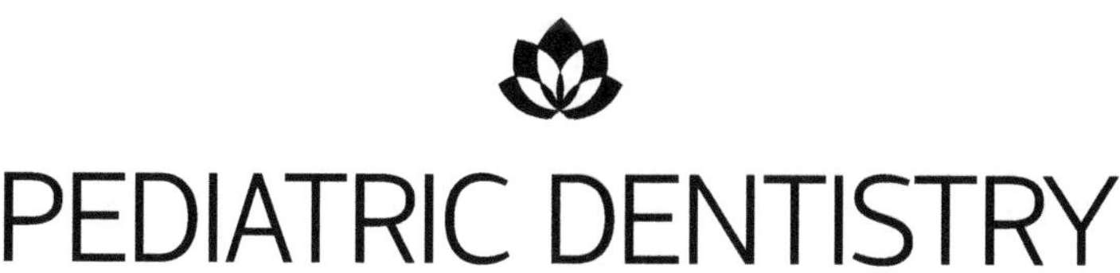

PEDIATRIC DENTISTRY

"Predicting the future isn't magic, it's artificial intelligence."
DaveWaters

In a study in 2017, automated tooth detection and numbering was conducted by a CNN that used a heuristic method to detect teeth. [9] Advances in the teeth detection field have led to heuristic techniques, thereby significantly increasing the accuracy of tooth shape determination[10]. AI has numerous potential applications which would change the face of behavioral pediatric practice in future. AI enabled restorative dentistry with computer-aided design and manufacturing would emerge a boon to pediatric restorations in terms of time and aesthetics.

In the mixed dentition period, the sizes of unerupted premolars and canines can be predicted using ANN. (15) AI enabled pain control gadgets is the new, smarter way towards injection-free pedodontics practice. The various 4D goggles, movies, animations and virtual reality-based games can be used as a behavior modification aid for pediatric patients(128).

CHAPTER TEN

ORAL AND MAXILLOFACIAL SURGERY

"The techniques of artificial intelligence are to the mind what bureaucracy is to human social interaction."

TerryWinograd

Other ingenious applications of AI include "bioprinting" where living tissue and even organs can be constructed in consecutive thin layers of cells which in the future may be used for reconstruction of oral hard and soft tissues lost due to pathological or accidental reasons and robotic surgery, where robotic surgeons perform semi-automated surgical tasks with increasing efficiency under the guidance of an expert surgeon.(5)

AI software programs has helps in planning surgeries by preserving the vital structures around to the smallest detail before the actual surgery with higher intra operative accuracy. One progressive clinical application is image guided surgery that admit further accurate surgical resection thereby decreasing need for revision procedures. The enormous use of artificial intelligence in oral and maxillofacial surgery is alongside the evolution of robotic surgery where human body motion and human intelligence is simulated(44)

A comparative study conducted by Raphael Patcas et al. on facial attractiveness between artificial-intelligence based scoring and conventional rater group in cleft patients uncovered equivalent outcomes among them(44). It introduces an ovel method in dentistry to rate facial attractiveness, by a face detector and a dedicated CNN (Convolutional Neural Networks). This study made it evident that the presented AI-based scoring is in need of further perfection and refinement to differentiate cleft features of the face that negatively influencethe human perception of attractiveness.

The tremendous utilization of artificial intelligence in oral and maxillofacial surgery is alongside the evolution of robotic surgery where human body motion and human intelligence is simulated.

CHAPTER ELEVEN

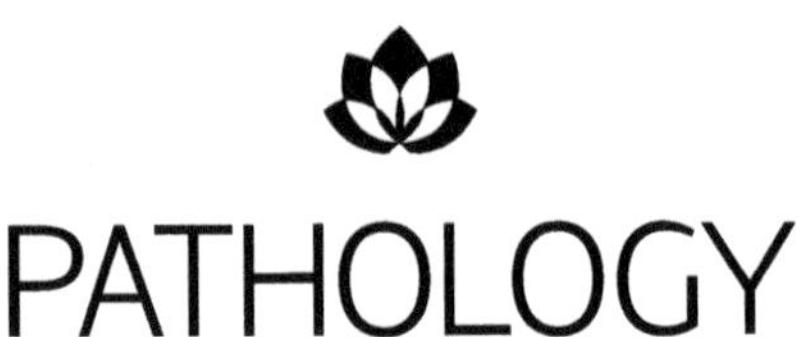

PATHOLOGY

"Is artificial intelligence less than our intelligence?"
SpikeJonze

Microscopic morphology is taken into account the gold standard in diagnostic pathology. Pathology specimens undergo multiple processes that include formalin fixation, grossing, paraffin embedding, tissue sectioning and at last staining. In general, it's human pathologist who gives pathology diagnosis by analyzing the specimen. However, the main limitation related to morphologic diagnosis is that the variability among the pathologists. In this way, for predictable and progressively precise conclusion, it is imperative to present AI in the pathology space. Further the need of computer-aided image classification system with quantitative analysis of histological features for rapid, consistent and quantitative diagnosis is necessary(129).

In a study, an open decision-support system based on Bayes' theorem connected to a relational database was developed using the C++ programming language. The software was tested in the computerisation of a surgical pathology service and in simulating the diagnosis of 43 known cases of oral bone disease. The simulation was performed after the system was initially filled with data from 401 cases of oral bone disease. Combining a relational database and an open decision-support system in the same user-friendly environment proved effective in simulating diagnoses based on information from an updated database.(130)

CHAPTER TWELVE

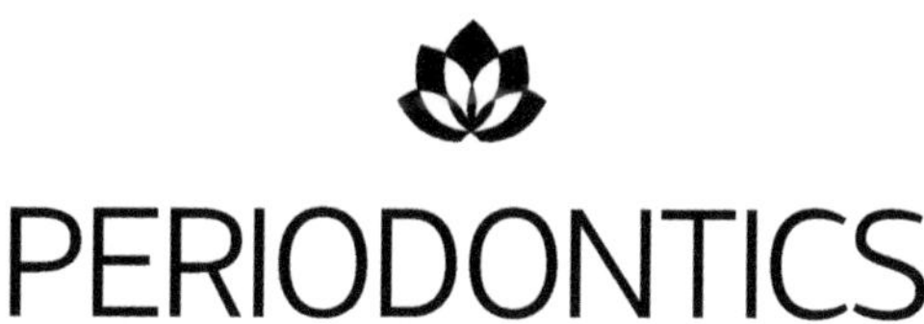

PERIODONTICS

"The countries with the highest robot density have among the lowest unemployment rates.
Technology and humans combined in the right way will drive prosperity."
Ulrich Spiesshofer

Deep learning analysis using radiographs can help in diagnosing and treatment planning of periodontal diseases by the early detection of periodontal changes(131), bone loss, and changes in bone density and detection of periimplantitis.(132) This helps in early intervention in implantology. ANN (Artificial Neural Network) can also effectively be used in classifying patients into aggressive periodontitis and chronic periodontitis group based on their immune response profile(133).

In a study by J.F. Farzad et al. age, sex, probing pocket depth, clinical attachment loss, and plaque index were selected as the main variables in neural network learning for the diagnosis of periodontal disease. Artificial neural networks have been used to help physicians in diseases diagnosis for the past five decades.(133)

Early prediction of gum disease helps to cure the tooth loss problem. Artificial Intelligent techniques are indeed worth exploring or diagnosis & prediction of complex medical problems. In a study by Thakur A. et al., a feed forward neural network with back propagation was used for prediction of possibility of periodontal and gingivitis gen diseases is estimated from symptoms and risk factors given by the patients.(134) Nakano Y. et al., presented an effective method of classifying oral malodor from oral microbiota in saliva by using a support vector machine (SVM), an artificial neural network (ANN). And a decision tree.(135) This approach uses concentrations of methyl mercaptan in mouth air as an indicator of oral malodor, and peak areas of terminal restriction fragment (T-RF) length polymorphisms (T-RFLPs)of the 16S ¡RNA gene as data for supervised machine-learning methods, without identifying specific species producing oral malodorous compounds. 16SrRNA genes were amplified from saliva samples from 309 subjects, and T-RFLP analysis was carried out with the DNA fragments. T-RFLP analysis provides information on microbiota consisting of fragment lengths and peak areas corresponding to bacterial strains. The peak area is equivalent to the frequency of a specific fragment when one molecule is selected from terminal fragments. The proportion that trained VM expressed as entropy achieved the highest classification accuracy, with a sensitivity of 51.1% and specificity of 95.0%. The AN and decision tree provided lower classification accuracies, and only classification by the ANN was improved by weighting with entropy from the frequency of appearance in samples, which increased the accuracy to 81.9% with a sensitivity of 60.2% and a specificity of 90.5%. The decision tree showed low classification accuracy under all conditions. Using T-RF proportions and frequencies, models to classify the presence of methylmercaptan, a volatile sulfur-containing compound that causes oral malodor, were developed. SVM classifiers successfully classified the presence of methylmercaptan with high specificity, and this classification is expected to be useful for screening saliva for oral malodor before visits to specialist clinics.

CHAPTER THIRTEEN

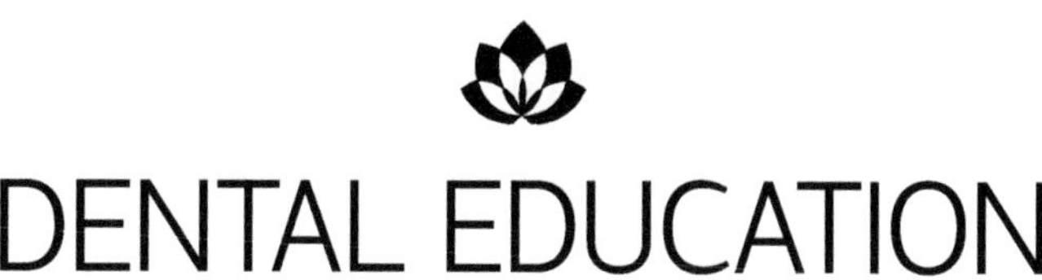

DENTAL EDUCATION

"If you don't have an AI strategy, you are going to dien the world that's coming."

Devin Wenig CEO, eBay CEO

Since its inception in the 1980s, the field of intelligent tutoring systems has come a long way. Both these systems, augmented reality and virtual reality are being used widely in the field of dental education to create situations that simulate clinical work on patients and eliminate all the risks associated while training on a live patient.(134) With the recent incorporation of artificial intelligence in intelligent tutoring systems like in the Unified Medical Language System (UMLS); there is a huge improvement in the quality of feedback that the preclinical virtual patient provides the students.(135,136)

The interactive interphase allows the students to evaluate their work and compare it to the ideal thus creating high-quality training environments. A number of studies carried out on the efficacy of these systems have indicated that students attain a competency based skill level at a faster rate than with traditional simulator units.(137,121) Clinical dentistry is a major part of dentistry for learning the skills and to enhance patient care.Traditionally,pre-clinical operative training for dental students is combination of theoretical teaching and practical learning. augmented and virtual reality has been incorporated into tutoring intelligent education system and training in dentistry [8]. These technologies enable simulation of the practical procedures in three dimensions and allows access to clinical and surgical techniques. The practice sessions can be done several time still the students get trained over the subject prior to actual handling of realclinical cases reducing the risk of iatrogenic error.(15)

CHAPTER FOURTEEN

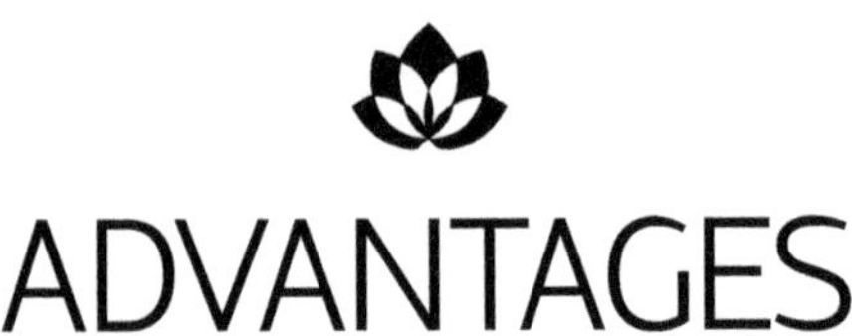

ADVANTAGES

"Artificial intelligence is a tool, not a threat."
Rodney Brooks

It made the dental treatments affordable, efficient and personalized. Dentists will be able to pin point specific problems thereby speeding the recovery. Tireless performance of the tasks which will save time(14) and provide patients accurate diagnosis. It helped the healthcare professionals to analyse and deliver informations more effectively than the human assistants and could overcome the communication gap. Alongwith images obtained from X-ray machines, they will be able to get preliminary analysis of those images.

Logical and feasible decisions without any involvement of human emotions which results in an accurate diagnosis(22) It provides standardization of procedures (38) It is an effective tool or aid to recognize patterns, predict events, and for grouping objects,eg.identify patients most at risk of missing appointments, precision scheduling, and empower individually tailored examination protocols (12) There has been a significant up take of these technologies in medicine, too, so far mainly in the field of computer vision. Diagnostic imaging is central in many healthcare fields, with AI being especially suitable to overcome the variability in subjective individual examination and to increase the effectiveness of care while lowering costs by eliminating routine tasks.

Digital health data are ubiquitously collected, and while so far these data are rather heterogenous, organizations are increasingly striving to provide cleaned, curated, and structured data. AI allows to integrate different and heterogenous data domains, for example, medical/dental history, socio-demographic and clinical data, imagery data, biomolecular data, social network data, etc., thereby making the best use of these multi-level data and allowing to grasp their interaction. AI facilitates research and discovery, by adding in silico experimentation options to conventional research hierarchies, complementing other research levels and existing modeling strategies.

As discussed, AI may streamline routine work and increase the face-to-face time doctors/dentists and their patients have ("humanizing care"). This may not only come via diagnostic assistance systems, but voice, speech, and text recognition and translation, enabling doctors/dentists to reduce time for record keeping. AI also promises to make healthcare more participatory, especially if patients provide their data actively, for example using wearables, etc. Patients will be empowered by self-monitoring and self-management.

Using these continuously collected data may also overcome the disadvantages of "on-off-medicine", where patients are seen only for a few minutes, while most health conditions are usually acquired over years, and come and go in (often times escalating) intervals (e.g.,periodontal disease).Continuous non-invasive monitoring of health and behavior will enable a much deeper, individual understanding of the drivers and processes underlying health and disease. Diagnostic and treatment costs may be decreased, thereby relieving healthcare systems burdened by an ageing society with an increasingly high numbers of complex, chronically ill cases. AI may also help to address shortages in work force, as observed and expected to continue in many parts of the globe, there by supporting to reach the World Health Organization (WHO)'s Sustainable Development Goals

CHAPTER FIFTEEN

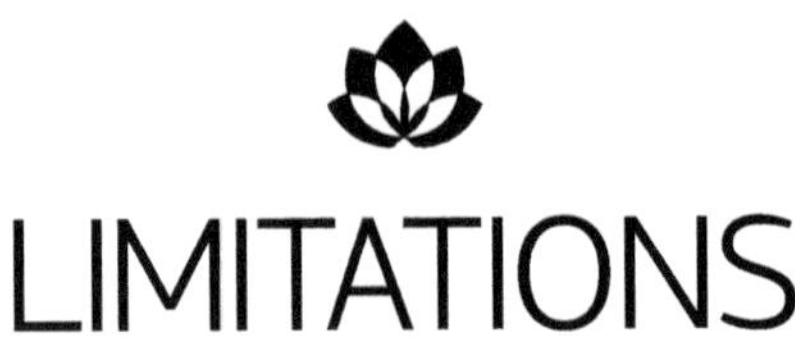

LIMITATIONS

"A computer would deserve to be called intelligent if it could deceive a human into believing that it was human."
Alan Turing

The system can never replace human expertise as humans are required to frequently monitor and update systems. Machines will require regular maintenance, and the cost to fix the setup would be high. Machines may be able to store a large amount of data but can never be compared to the human brain. Also, Machines would not be able to alter their responses in changing situations as they function in the manner they are programmed. Human beings are emotional intellectuals and can think, feel and use their senses to come to a solution. But the major disadvantage of a machine is that they lack empathy and care.

Despite all the potential, AI solutions have largely not entered routine medical practice. In dentistry, for example, convolutional NNs have only been adopted in research settings from 2015 onwards, mainly on dental radiographs, and the first applications involving these technologies are now entering the clinical arena. This is all the more surprising when acknowledging that dentistry is especially suited to applying AI tasks:

1) In dentistry, imagery plays an important role and is the cornerstone of most patients' dental voyage, from screening to treatment planning and conduct.

2) Dentistry regularly uses different imagery materials from the same anatomical region of the same individual, regularly accompanied by non-imagery data like clinical records and general and dental history data, including systemic conditions and medications. Moreover, data are often

collected over multiple time points. AI is suited to integrate and cross-link these data effectively and improve diagnostics, prediction, and decision-making.

3) Many dental conditions (caries, apical lesions, periodontal bone loss) are relatively prevalent. Building up datasets with a high number of "affected" cases can be managed with limited efforts.

There are three main reasons why dentistry has not yet fully adopted AI technologies. Tackling these reasons will help to make dental AI technologies better and facilitate their uptake in clinical care.

First, medical and dental data are not as available and accessible as other data due to data protection concerns and organizational hurdles. Data are often locked within segregated, individualized, and limitedly interoperable systems. Datasets lack structure and are often relatively small, at least when compared with other datasets in the AI realm. Data on each patient are complex, multi-dimensional, and sensitive, with limited options for triangulating or validating them. Medical and dental data, for example, from electronic medical records, show low variable completeness, with data of ten missing systematically and not at random. Sampling often leads to selection bias, with either overly sick (e.g., hospital data), overly healthy (e.g., data collected by wearable devices), or overly affluent (e.g., data from those who afford dental care in countries lacking universal healthcare coverage) individuals being over-represented. AI applications developed on such data will be inherently biased.

Second, processing data and measuring and validating results are often insufficiently replicable and robust in dental AI research. It remains unclear how datasets were selected, curated, and preprocessed. Data is often used for training and testing, leading to "data snooping bias." It is usually impossible to define a "hard" gold standard, and there is no agreement on how many experts are required to label a data point and how to merge different labels of such"fuzzy" gold standards.

Third, the outcomes of AI indentistry are often not readily applicable: The single information provided by most of today's dental AI applications will only partially inform the required and complex decision-making in clinical care. Moreover, questions toward responsibilities and transparency remain.

CHAPTER SIXTEEN

FUTURE ADVANCEMENTS

"Anything that could give rise to smarter-than-human intelligence — in the form of Artificial Intelligence, brain-computer interfaces, or neuroscience-based human intelligence enhancement — wins hands down beyond contest as doing the most to change the world. Nothing else is even in the same league."
Eliezer Yudkowsky

As AI advances, it may result in an overall better healthcare experience by way of readily accessible, intelligible, and actionable data. This will undoubtedly lead to a reduction in downstream medical costs as technology-based diagnostics and treatment plans spur upfront payments minus delay, inefficiency, and human error such as over-diagnosis, under-diagnosis, and misdiagnosis. AI will also open the door to unified treatment options among multiline carriers and integration of medical data across various healthcare fields. As data-driven treatment becomes more common place, medical disciplines will inevitably begin to overlap until dental and healthcare integration is complete. When diagnostics and treatment are isolated to a single branch of medicine, complications can occur, or, at the very least, a patient may not get the treatment that's best for them. In dental care, one of the biggest road blocks to efficiency and quality assurance is simply not having enough information about the patient. Not only can this slow down the claims process, but it also can keep dentists from doing their job to the best of their ability. AI is posed to overcome such hurdles by simply integrating all available data into its algorithmic program and providing output specific to the medical field and request. This will play a major role in off setting liability and in protecting dentists, patients, and insurers as well.

Research and development is currently underway in AI predictive analytics capable of utilizing ML, DL, and computer vision to create future-based diagnoses of pathologies and conditions.Whereas medicine currently relies on professional "guesstimates" to determine future outcomes, there is no technological basis on which we can, with certainty and accuracy, build those prognosis.

But what if, as a dentist, you could run an image of your patient's teeth and gums through an AI program and know with near-certainty that in precisely six months, their tooth decay will become untreatable and require a crown? And while a human dentist may be able to perform a similar parlor trick, AI will hardly be guessing. Instead, it will be using millions of data points to make a highly informed, educated, and quantified projection down to afraction of a percentile. Predictive diagnostics will also serve as grounds for insurance claim authorization, aiding in preventive care that keeps patients healthy instead of simply treating the disease. With networked AI among clinics and insurers, pre-authorization may even occur in real time, and patients can enjoy same-day diagnosis, authorization, and treatment. A combination of predictive diagnostics, insurance fraud detection, and automated underwriting may involve the simple tap of a button and an immediate response.

AI will also give clout to research being conducted on the connection between periodontal diseases and common illnesses such as diabetes and hypertension. With medical and dental integration, dentistry will enjoy new found support in healthcare and much needed standardization of care that enhances clinical capabilities and simply let dentists do their job.

CHAPTER SEVENTEEN

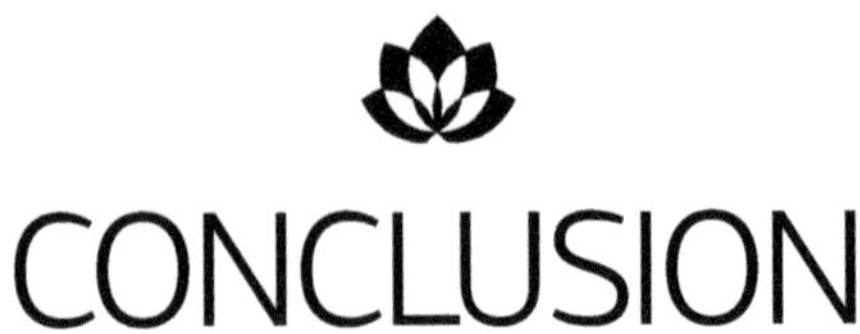

CONCLUSION

"Machine intelligence is the last invention that humanity will ever need to make."
Nick Bostrom

Applications of AI in everyday life are growing leaps and bounds. Dentists have always been at the forefront of implementing a technology. Hence, understanding the various concepts and the techniques involved will have a clear advantage in the future when it is time to adapt to the change with redefined roles for a rewarding practice.(22) There are so many techniques that are being used in artificial intelligence and it is still in its budding stage. The prevailing researches have provided sufficient evidence of its efficacy. There is a common notion that artificial intelligence will replace the clinicians, which is why they have been quite skeptical in embracing it. As a matter of fact, the incorporation of these techniques will not only increase the efficiency of the specialists but also help in better patient care. It needs to be understood that artificial intelligence has been given birth by humans, therefore, it will never be able to enslave them in unfamiliar situations unless trained to doso.(14)

The next decade will prove if this time the expectations for tangible AI applications are met by actual outcomes or if once again an AI-winter buries hopes and excitement. In particular in healthcare, the stakes are high. There is reasonable concern about data protection and data security and about handing over critical medical decisions to computers. However, AI has the potential to revolutionize healthcare and, with it, dentistry; AI may assist in addressing the weaknesses harshly criticized in conventional dental care (Wattetal.2019). Dentistry and, specifically, dental research, has a role to ensure that AI will make dental care better, at lower costs, to the benefit of patients, providers, and the wider society.

References

1. Tandon D, Rajawat J. Present and future of artificial intelligence in dentistry. J Oral Biol Craniofacial Res. 2020;10(4):391–6.
2. Chen YW, Stanley K, Att W. Artificial intelligence in dentistry: Current applications and future perspectives. Quintessence Int (Berl). 2020;51(3):248–57.
3. McCarthy J. Artificial Intelligence, Logic and Formalizing Common Sense. Philos Log Artif Intell. 1989;161–90.
4. Feigenbaum MJ, Mermin ND. Vol.56, American Journal of Physics. 1988.18–21p.
5. Tauqir S. Is Artificial Intelligence Transforming Dentistry Today? J Gandhara Med Dent Sci. 2021;8(4):1.
6. Cohen PR, Feigenbaum EA, Barr A. The handbook of artificial intelligence. Volume III. 2014;II:659.
7. Kohn MK, Berta W, Langley A, Davis D. Evidence-based decision making in healthcare settings: From theory to practice. Vol. 11, Advances in Health Care Management. 2011.p.215–34.
8. Albus JS. Outline for a theory of intelligence. IEEE Trans Syst Man Cybern. 1991;21(3):473–509.
9. Zackova E. Intelligence Explosion Quest for Human kind. 2015;31–43.
10. Ahmed N, Abbasi MS, Zuberi F, Qamar W, Halim MS Bin, Maqsood A, et al. Artificial Intelligence Techniques: Analysis, Application, and Outcome in Dentistry – A Systematic Review. Biomed Res Int. 2021;2021.
11. Bansod AV, Pisulkar SK. Artificial Intelligence & Its Contemporary Applications in Dentistry. 2021;12(6):4192–6.
ARTIFICIALINTELLIGENCEINDENTISTRY 135
12. Msungu P, Mlangwa M, Sohal KS. Self-perceived Satisfaction with Dental Appearance and Associated Factors among Secondary School Students in Iringa, Tanzania.J Dent Res Rev 2021;8:97–101.
13. Rajaraman V. John McCarthy- Father of artificial intelligence. Resonance. 2014;19(3):198–207.
14. Alexander B, John S. Artificial Intelligence in Dentistry: Current Concepts and a Peep Into the Future. Int J Adv Res.2018;6(12):1105–8.
15. J Kurup R, Sodhi A, R S. Dentistry and Artificial Intelligence. Acta Sci Dent Scienecs. 2020;4(10):26–32.

16. Schwendicke F, Samek W, Krois J. Artificial Intelligence in Dentistry: Chances and Challenges. J Dent Res. 2020;99(7):769–74.
17. Katne T, Kanaparthi A, Gotoor S, Muppirala S, Devaraju R, Gantala R. Artificial Intelligence: Demystifying Dentistry – The Future and Beyond. Int J Contemp Med Surg Radiol. 2019;4(4):6–9.
18. Wulff A, Montag S, Steiner B, Marschollek M, Beerbaum P, Karch A, et al. CADDIE2- evaluation of a clinical decision- support system for early detection of systemic inflammatory response syndrome in paediatric intensive care: study protocol for a diagnostic study. BMJ Open. 2019;9(6):1–5.
19. Artificial intelligence: contemporary applications and future compass
20. Bahaa K, Noor G, Yousif Y. The Artificial Intelligence Approach for Diagnosis, Treatment and Modelling in Orthodontic. Princ Contemp Orthod. 2011
21. Wulff A, Montag S, Steiner B, Marschollek M, Beerbaum P, Karch A, et al. CADDIE2- evaluation of a clinical decision- support system for early detection of systemic inflammatory response syndrome in paediatric intensive care: study protocol for a diagnostic study. BMJ Open. 2019;9(6).
22. Brickley MR, Shepherd JP, Armstrong RA. Neural networks: A new technique for development of decision support systems in dentistry. J Dent.1998;26(4):305–9.
ARTIFICIALINTELLIGENCEINDENTISTRY 136
23. Steimann F. On the use and usefulness of fuzzy sets in medical AI. Artif Intell Med. 2001;21(1–3):131–7.
24. Ramesh AN, Kambhampati C, Monson JRT, Drew PJ. Artificial intelligence in medicine. Ann R Coll Surg Engl.2004;86(5):334–8.
25. Kassianos AP, Emery JD, Murchie P, Walter FM. Smart phone applications for melanoma detection by community, patient and generalist clinician users: A review. Br J Dermatol. 2015;172(6):1507–18.
26. Buchanan JA. Experience with Virtual Reality- Based Technology in Teaching Restorative Dental Procedures. J Dent Educ. 2004;68(12):1258–65.
27. Dutã M, Amariei C. An overview of virtual and augmented reality in dental education. J Oral Heal Dent Manag.2011;10(1):42–9.
28. Kikuchi H, Ikeda M, Araki K. Evaluation of a Virtual Reality Simulation System for Porcelain Fused to Metal Crown Preparation at Tokyo Medical and Dental University. J Dent Educ.2013;77(6):782–92.
29. Wiederhold MD, Gao K, Wiederhold BK. Clinical use of virtual reality

distraction system to reduce anxiety and pain in dental procedures. Cyberpsychology, Behav Soc Netw. 2014;17(6):359–65.

30. Mijwel MM. History of Artificial Intelligence Yapay Zekânın T arihi. Comput Sci. 2015;(April2015):3–4.

31. Gupta R, Tanwar S, Al-Turjman F, Italiya P, Nauman A, Kim SW. Smart Contract Privacy Protection Using AI in Cyber-Physical Systems: Tools, Techniques and Challenges. IEEE Access. 2020;8:24746–72.

32. Lazarus-Karaoglan T. Medical electronics. IEEE Spectr. 1999;36(1):79–83.

33. Vijai C, Wisetsri W. Rise of Artificial Intelligence in Healthcare Startups in India. Adv Manag. 2021;14(1):48–52.

34. Yaji A, Prasad S, Oxford T, Institutions E, Deficiency VD. Artificial Intelligence in
ARTIFICIALINTELLIGENCEINDENTISTRY 137
Dento-Maxillofacial Radiology ACTA SCIENTIFIC DENTAL SCIENCES (ISSN : 2581-4893) Artificial Intelligence in Dento-Maxillofacial Radiology. 2019;(October).

35. Saghiri MA, Asgar K, Boukani KK, Lotfi M, Aghili H, Delvarani A, et al. A new approach for locating the minor apical foramen using an artificial neural network. Int Endod J. 2012;45(3):257–65.

36. Chen YC, Hong D, Wu CW, Mupparapu M. The use of deep convolutional neural networks in biomedical imaging: A review. J Orofac Sci. 2019;11(1):3–10.

37. Dar-Odeh NS, Alsmadi OM, Bakri F, Abu-Hammour Z, Shehabi AA, Al-Omiri MK, et al. Predicting recurrent aphthous ulceration using genetic algorithms-optimized neural networks. Adv Appl Bioinforma Chem. 2010;3(1):7–13.

38. Kalappanavar A, Sneha S, Annigeri RG. Artificial intelligence : A dentist's
perspective. 2018;5:2–4.

39. Hu XS, Nascimento TD, Bender MC, Hall T, Petty S, O'Malley S, et al. Feasibility of a real-time clinical augmented reality and artificial intelligence framework for pain detection and localization from the brain. J Med Internet Res.2019;21(6):1–11.

40. Wang CW, Huang CT, Lee JH, Li CH, Chang SW, Siao MJ, et al. A benchmark for comparison of dental radiography analysis algorithms. Med Image Anal. 2016;31:63–76.

41. Tan MS, Tan JW, Chang SW, Yap HJ, Kareem SA, Zain RB. A genetic

programming approach to oral cancer prognosis. Peer J. 2016;2016(9):1–15.
42. Scrobotă I, Băciuţ G, Filip AG, Todor B, Blaga F, Băciuţ MF. Application of fuzzy
Logic in oral cancer risk assessment. Iran J Public Health.2017;46(5):612–9.
43. Papantonopoulos G, Takahashi K, Bountis T, Loos BG. Artificial neural networks for the diagnosis of aggressive periodontitis trained by immunologic parameters. PLoS One.2014;9(3):1–7.
44. Patcas R, Timofte R, Volokitin A, Agustsson E, Eliades T, Eichenberger M, et al. Facial attractiveness of cleft patients: A direct comparison between artificial-intelligence-based scoring and conventional rater groups. Eur J Orthod. 2019;41(4):428–33.

45. Patcas R, Bernini DAJ, Volokitin A, Agustsson E, Rothe R, Timofte R. Applying artificial intelligence to assess the impact of orthognathic treatment on facial attractiveness and estimated age. Int J Oral Maxillofac Surg. 2019;48(1):77–83.
46. Sami T, Al H. Personal Identification System Using Dental Panoramic Radiograph Based on Meta_Heuristic Algorithm Personal Identification System Using Dental Panoramic Radiograph Based on Meta_ Heuristic Algorithm. 2019;14(April):344–50.
47. Ehtesham H, Safdari R, Mansourian A, Tahmasebian S, Mohammadzadeh N, Ghazisaeedi M, et al. Clinical decision support system, a potential solution for diagnostic accuracy improvement in oral squamous cell carcinoma: A systematic review. J Oral Heal Oral Epidemiol. 2017;6(4):187–95.
48. Tang A, Tam R, Cadrin-Chênevert A, Guest W, Chong J, Barfett J, et al. Canadian Association of Radiologists White Paper on Artificial Intelligence in Radiology. Can Assoc Radiol J. 2018;69(2):120–35.
49. De Tobel J, Radesh P, Vandermeulen D, Thevissen PW. An automated technique to stage lower third molar development on panoramic radiographs for ageestimation: A pilot study. J Forensic Odontostomatol. 2017;35(2):42–54.
50. Lehmann TM, Gröndahl HG, Benn DK. Computer-based registration for digital subtraction indental radiology. Dentomaxillofacial Radiol. 2000;29(6):323–46.
51. Bossuyt PM, Irwig L, Craig J, Glasziou P. Comparative accuracy: Assessing new tests agains texisting diagnostic pathways. Br Med J.

2006;332(7549):1089–92.
52. Alkasab TK, Bizzo BC, Berland LL, Nair S, Pandharipande P V., Harvey HB. Creation of an Open Framework for Point-of-Care Computer-Assisted Reporting and Decision Support Tools for Radiologists. J Am Coll Radiol. 2017;14(9):1184–9.
53. Gillies RJ, Kinahan PE, Hricak H. Radiomics: Images are more than pictures, they are data Radiology. 2016;278(2):563–77.
54. Zalis M, Harris M. Advanced search of the electronic medical record: Augmenting safety and efficiency in radiology. J Am Coll Radiol. 2010;7(8):625–33.
55. Tran K, Bøtker JP, Aframian A, Memarzadeh K. Artificial intelligence for medical
ARTIFICIALINTELLIGENCEINDENTISTRY 139
Imaging [Internet]. Artificial Intelligence in Healthcare. INC; 2020.143–162p.
56. Wenzel A. Computer-Automated Caries Detection in Digital Bitewings: Consistency of a Program and Its Influence on Observer Agreement. Caries Res. 2001;35(1):12–20.
57. Farman AG, Vandre RH, Webber RL. Future trends in dental radiology. Oral Surgery, Oral Med Oral Pathol Oral Radiol. 1995; 80(4):471–8.
58. Zhang H, Ong SH, Foong KWC, Dhar T. Dimensional Orthodontics Visualization System With Dental Study Models and Orthopantomograms. 2005;768–87.
59. Gerlach NL, Meijer GJ, Kroon DJ, Bronkhorst EM, Bergé SJ, Maal TJJ. Evaluation of the potential of automatic segmentation of the mandibular canal using cone-beam computed tomography.Br J Oral Maxillo fac Surg. 2014;52(9):838–44.
60. Tassoker M. Prediction of Osteoporosis Through Deep Learning Algorithms on Panoramic Radiographs. 2022;1–14.
61. Kavitha MS, Asano A, Taguchi A, Heo MS. The combination of a histogram-based clustering algorithm and support vector machine for the diagnosis of osteoporosis. Imaging Sci Dent. 2013;43(3):153–61.
62. Kavitha MS, Kumar PG, Park SY, Huh KH, Heo MS, KuritaT, et al. Automatic detection of osteoporosis based on hybrid genetic swarm fuzzy classifier approaches. Dentomaxillofacial Radiol. 2016;45(7).
63. Strut analysis for osteoporosis detection model using dental panoramic radiography-Pub Med [Internet]. [cited2022Mar23].
64. Bormane DDS, Kakkeri RB. Detection of Temporo mandibular Joint

Disorder Using Surface Electromypgraphy by Supervised Classification Models.
65. Bas B, Ozgonenel O, Ozden B, Bekcioglu B, Bulut E, Kurt M. Use of artificial neural network in differentiation of subgroups of temporo mandibular internal derangements: A preliminary study. J Oral Maxillofac Surg. 2012;70(1):51–9.
66. Orhan K, Driesen L, Shujaat S, Jacobs R, Chai X. Development and Validation of a Magnetic Resonance Imaging-Based Machine Learning Model for TMJ Pathologies.
ARTIFICIALINTELLIGENCEINDENTISTRY 140
Biomed Res Int.2021;2021.
67. Kim D, Choi E, Jeong HG, Chang J, Youm S. Expert system for mandibular condyle detection and osteoarthritis classification in panoramic imaging using r-cnn and cnn. Appl Sci. 2020;10(21):1–10.
68. Jabbar SI, Day CR, Heinz N, Chadwick EK. Using Convolutional Neural Network for edge detection in musculoskeletal ultrasound images. Proc Int Jt Conf Neural Networks. 2016;2016-Octob:4619–26.
69. Jung SK, Lim HK, Lee S, Cho Y, Song IS. Deep active learning for automatic segmentation of maxillary sinus lesions using a convolutional neural network. Diagnostics. 2021;11(4):1–11.
70. Limonadi FM, McCartney S, Burchiel KJ. Design of an artificial neural network for diagnosis of facial pain syndromes. Stereo tact Funct Neuro surg. 2006;84(5–6):212–20.
71. Rioux-Forker D, Deziel AC, Williams LS, Muzaffar AR. Odontogenic Cysts and Tumors. Ann Plast Surg. 2019 Apr;82(4):469–77.
72. Mikulka J, Gescheidtová E, Kabrda M, Peřina V. Classification of jaw bone cysts and necrosis via the processing of ortho pantomograms. Radio engineering. 2013;22(1):114–22.
73. Rana M, Modrow D, Keuchel J, Chui C, Rana M, Wagner M, et al. Development and evaluation of an automatic tumor segmentation tool: A comparison between automatic, semi-automatic and manual segmentation of mandibular odontogenic cysts and tumors. J Cranio-Maxillofacial Surg [Internet]. 2015;43(3):355–9.
74. López F, Rodrigo JP, Silver CE, HaigentzJr M, Bishop JA, Strojan P, et al. Cervical lymph node metastases from remote primary tumor sites. Head Neck[Internet]. 2015/12/29.2016Apr;38Suppl1(Suppl1):E2374–85.
75. Dohopolski M, Chen L, Sher DJ, Wang J. Predicting Lymph Node Metastasis in Patients with Oropharyngeal Cancer by Convolutional Neural

Networks with associated Epistemic Uncertainty. Int J Radiat Oncol [Internet]. 2019;105(1):S122.

76. Ariji Y, Sugita Y, Nagao T, Nakayama A, Fukuda M, Kise Y, et al. CT evaluation of extranodal extension of cervical lymph node metastases in patients with oral squamous cell carcinoma using deep learning classification. Oral Radiol [Internet].2020;36(2):148–
ARTIFICIALINTELLIGENCEINDENTISTRY 141
55.

77. Yardimci G, Kutlubay Z, Engin B, Tuzun Y. Precancerous lesions of oral mucosa. World J Clin cases [Internet]. 2014Dec16;2(12):866–72.

78. Maghsoudi R, Bagheri A, Maghsoudi MT. Diagnosis Prediction of Lichen Planus, Leukoplakia and Oral Squamous Cell Carcinoma by using an Intelligent System Based on Artificial Neural Networks. J Dentomaxillofacial Radiol Pathol Surg. 2013;2(2):1–8.

79. Khanagar SB, Naik S, Al Kheraif AA, Vishwanathaiah S, Maganur PC, Alhazmi Y, et al. Application and performance of artificial intelligence technology in oral cancer diagnosis and prediction of prognosis: A systematic review. Diagnostics. 2021;11(6):1–12.

80. García-Pola M, Pons-Fuster E, Suárez-Fernández C, Seoane-Romero J, Romero-Méndez A, López-Jornet P. Role of artificial intelligence in the early diagnosis of oral cancer.A scoping review.Cancers (Basel). 2021;13(18):1–25.

81. Song B, Sunny S, Uthoff RD, Patrick S, Suresh A, Kolur T, et al. Automatic classification of dual-modalilty, smartphone-based oral dysplasia and malignancy images using deep learning. Biomed Opt Express. 2018;9(11):5318.

82. Tanriver G, Soluk Tekkesin M, Ergen O. Automated detection and classification of oral lesions using deep learning to detect oral potentially malignant disorders. Cancers (Basel). 2021;13(11).

83. Shamim M, Syed S, Shiblee M, Usman M, Ali S. Automated detection of oral pre-cancerous tongue lesions using deep learning for early diagnosis of oral cavity cancer.:1–25.

84. Jeyaraj PR, Samuel Nadar ER. Computer-assisted medical image classification for early diagnosis of oral cancer employing deep learning algorithm. J Cancer Res Clin Oncol [Internet]. 2019;145(4):829–37.

85. Poedjiastoeti W, Suebnukarn S. Application of Convolutional Neural Network in the Diagnosis of Jaw Tumors. 2018;24(3):236–41.

86. Van Staveren HJ, Van Veen RLP, Speelman OC, Witjes MJH, Star WM,

Roodenburg JLN. Classification of clinical auto fluorescence spectra of oral leukoplakia using an
ARTIFICIALINTELLIGENCEINDENTISTRY 142
artificial neural network: A pilot study.Oral Oncol. 2000;36(3):286–93.
87. Vigneswaran N, Kang SK, Niederman R, Christodoulides NJ. Nuclear F-actin Cytology in Oral Epithelial Dysplasia and Oral Squamous Cell Carcinoma. 2020;
88. Shams WK, Htike ZZ. Oral Cancer Prediction Using Gene Expression Profiling and Machine Learning. 2017;12(15):4893–8.
89. Sharma N, Om H. Usage of Probabilistic and General Regression Neural Network for Early Detection and Prevention of Oral Cancer.2015.
90. Alawi F. Pigmented lesions of the oral cavity: an update. Dent Clin North Am. 2013/08/15.2013Oct; 57(4):699–710.
91. Phillips M, Marsden H, Jaffe W, Matin RN, Wali GN. Assessment of Accuracy of an Artificial Intelligence Algorithm to Detect Melanomain Images of Skin Lesions. 2019;2(10):1–12.
92. Liu G, Li Y, Zhang W, Zhang L. AI for Precision Medicine — Review A Brief Review of Artificial Intelligence Applications and Algorithms for Psychiatric Disorders. Engineering [Internet]. 2020;6(4):462–7.
93. Hagen E, Sømhovd M, Hesse M, Arnevik EA, Erga AH. Measuring cognitive impairment in young adults with poly substance use disorder with MoCA or BRIEF-A –The significance of psychiatric symptoms. J Subst AbuseTreat.2019Feb;97:21–7.
94. Barker LC, Gruneir A, Fung K, Herrmann N, Kurdyak P, Lin E, et al. Predicting psychiatric readmission: sex-specific models to predict 30-day readmission following acute psychiatric hospitalization. Soc Psychiatry Psychiatr Epidemiol. 2018Feb;53(2):139–49.
95. Shen C-C, Hu L-Y, Tsai S-J, Yang AC, Chen P-M, Hu Y-H. Risk stratification for the early diagnosis of border line personality disorder using psychiatric co-morbidities. Early Interv Psychiatry. 2018Aug;12(4):605–12.
96. Shaukat N, Ali DM, Razzak J. Physical and mental health impacts of COVID-19 on healthcare workers: a scoping review. Int J Emerg Med [Internet]. 2020;13(1):40.
ARTIFICIALINTELLIGENCEINDENTISTRY 143
97. Whiteside SPH, Gryczkowski MR, Biggs BK, Fagen R, Owusu D. Validation of the Spence Children's Anxiety Scale's obsessive compulsive sub scale in a clinical and community sample. J Anxiety Disord.

2012Jan;26(1):111–6.
98. Peng Z, Hu Q, Dang J. Multi-kernel SVM based depression recognition using social media data. Int J Mach Learn Cybern. 2019Jan 1;10.
99. Heinsfeld AS, Franco AR, Craddock RC, Buchweitz A, Meneguzzi F. Identification of autism spectrum disorder using deep learning and the ABIDE dataset. Neuro Image Clin [Internet]. 2017Aug30;17:16–23.
100. Hashimoto DA, Witkowski E, Gao L, Meireles O, Rosman G. Artificial intelligence in anesthesiology: Current techniques, clinical applications, and limitations. Anesthesiology. 2020;(Xxx):379–94.
101. Hassanzadeh P, Atyabi F, Dinarvand R. The significance of artificial intelligence in drug delivery system design. Adv Drug Deliv Rev. 2019;151–152:169–90.
102. Lv J, Deng S, Zhang L. A review of artificial intelligence applications for antimicrobial resistance. Biosaf Heal. 2021;3(1):22–31.
103. Devito KL, de Souza Barbosa F, Filho WNF. An artificial multilayer perceptron neural network for diagnosis of proximal dental caries. Oral Surgery, Oral Med Oral Pathol Oral Radiol Endodontology. 2008;106(6):879–84.
104. Bhan A, Goyal A, Harsh, Chauhan N, Wang CW. Feature Line profile based automatic detection of dental caries in bite wing radiography. Proc-2016 Int Conf Micro-Electronics Telecommun Eng ICMETE2016. 2016;(February2019):635–40.
105. Miladinović M, Mihailović B, Mladenović D, Duka M, Živković D, Mladenović S, et al. Veštačka inteligencija u kliničkoj medicine I stomatologiji. Vojnosanit Pregl. 2017;74(3):267–72.
106. Abastabar M, HaghaniI, Ahangarkani F, Rezai MS, Armaki MT, Roodgari S. Institutional Login. 2021;2019–21.
107. Rhienmora P, Gajananan K, Haddawy P, Dailey MN, Suebnukarn S. Augmented Reality Haptics System for Dental Surgical Skills Training. In: Proceedings of the 17th ACM Symposium on Virtual Reality Software and Technology [Internet]. New York, NY,

USA: Association for Computing Machinery; 2010. p. 97–98. (VRST '10).
108. Bhatia A, Singh R. Using Bayesian network as decision making system tool for deciding treatment plan for dental caries. J Acad Ind Res.2013 Jan1;2.
109. Albahbah A, El-Bakry H, Abdelghany S. A New Optimized Approach for Detection of Caries in Panoramic Images. Int J Comput Eng Inf Technol.

2016 Sep1;8:163–70.
110. Yin MS, Haddawy P, Suebnukarn S, Schultheis H, Rhienmora P. Use of haptic feedback to train correct application of force in endodontic surgery. Int Conf Intell User Interfaces,Proc IUI.2017Mar7;451–5.
111. Hammond P, Davenport JC, Fitzpatrick FJ. Logic-based integrity constraints and the design of dental prostheses. Artif Intell Med. 1993;5(5):431–46.
112. Vera V, Corchado E, Redondo R, Sedano J, García ÁE. Applying soft computing techniques to optimise a dental milling process. Neuro computing. 2013;109:94–104.
113. Vecsei B, Joós-Kovács G, Borbély J, Hermann P. Comparison of the accuracy of direct and indirect three-dimensional digitizing processes for CAD/CAM systems – An invitro study. J Prosthodont Res. 2017;61(2):177–84.
114. Deniz ST, Ozkan P, Ozkan G. The accuracy of the prediction models for surface roughness and micro hardness of denture teeth. Dent Mater J. 2019Dec;38(6):1012–8.
115. Li H, Lai L, Chen L, Lu C, Cai Q. The Prediction in Computer Color Matching of Dentistry Based on GA+BP Neural Network. Chen S, editor. Comput Math Methods Med [Internet]. 2015; 2015:816719.
116. Mine Y, Suzuki S, Eguchi T, Murayama T. Applying deep artificial neural network approach to maxillofacial prostheses coloration. J Prosthodont Res [Internet]. 2020;64(3):296–300.
117. Chen Q, Wu J, Li S, Lyu P, Wang Y, Li M. An ontology-driven, case-based clinical decision support model for removable partial denture design. Sci Rep [Internet]. 2016;6(1):27855.
ARTIFICIALINTELLIGENCEINDENTISTRY 145
118. Lim K, Moles DR, Downer MC, Speight PM. Opportunistic screening for oral cancer and precancer in general dental practice: Results of a demonstration study. Br Dent J. 2003;194(9):497–502.
119. Speight PM, Elliott AE, Jullien JA, Downer MC, Zakzrewska JM. The use of artificial intelligence to identify people at risk of oral cancer and precancer. Br Dent J. 1995;179(10):382–7.
120. Choudhary E, Vashisht A. Artificial Intelligence; Mutating Dentistry. Int J Res Anal Rev.2019;6(March):32–5.
121. Feeney L, Reynolds PA, Eaton KA, Harper J. A description of the new technologies used in transforming dental education. Br Dent J. 2008;204(1):19–28.

122. Kök H, Acilar AM, İzgi MS. Usage and comparison of artificial intelligence algorithms for determination of growth and development by cervical vertebrae stages in orthodontics. Prog Orthod. 2019;20(1).

123. Li P, Kong D, Tang T, Su D, Yang P, Wang H, et al. Orthodontic Treatment Planning based on Artificial Neural Networks. Sci Rep. 2019;9(1):1–9.

124. Sims-Williams JH, Brown ID, Matthewman A, Stephens CD. A computer-controlled expert system for orthodontic advice. Br Dent J. 1987;163(5):161–6.

125. Xie X, Wang L, Wang A. Artificial neural network modeling for deciding if extractions are necessary prior to orthodontic treatment. Angle Orthod. 2010;80(2):262–6.

126. Birnbaum NS, Aaronson HB. Dental impressions using 3D digital scanners: virtual becomes reality. Compend Contin Educ Dent. 2008;29(8):11–3.

127. Kattadiyil MT, Mursic Z, Alrumaih H, Goodacre CJ. Intraoral scanning of hard and soft tissues for partial removable dental prosthesis fabrication. J Prosthet Dent. 2014;112(3):444–8.

128. Dentistry P. Pedodontics and Preventive Dentistry. 2019;37(September): 31710003.

129. Narayan Biswal B, Narayan Das S, Kumar Das B, Rath R. Alteration of cellular
ARTIFICIALINTELLIGENCEINDENTISTRY 146
metabolism in cancer cells and its therapeutic. J oral Maxillofac Pathol. 2017;21(3):244–51.

130. Borra RC, Andrade PM, Corrêa L, Novelli MD. Development of an open case-based decision-support system for diagnosis in oral pathology. Eur J Dent Educ Off J Assoc Dent Educ Eur. 2007May;11(2):87–92.

131. Furman E, Roma Jasinewicius T, Bissada NF, Victoroff KZ, Skillicorn R, Buchner M.Virtual reality distraction for pain control during periodontal scaling and root planning procedures. J Am Dent Assoc. 2009;140(12):1508–16.

132. Sohmura T, Kusumoto N, Otani T, Yamada S, Wakabayashi K, Yatani H. CAD/CAM fabrication and clinical application of surgical template and bone model in oral implant surgery. Clin Oral Implants Res. 2009;20(1):87–93.

133. Papantonopoulos G, Takahashi K, Bountis T, Loos BG. Aggressive Periodontitis Defined by Recursive Partitioning Analysis of Immunologic

Factors. J Periodontol. 2013;84(7):974–84.
134. Murray T. Authoring Intelligent Tutoring Systems : An analysis of the state of theart To cite this version : HAL Id : hal-00197339 Authoring Intelligent Tutoring Systems : An Analysis of the State of the Art.2007
135. Crowley RS, Medvedeva O. An intelligent tutoring system for visual classification problem solving. Artif Intell Med. 2006;36(1):85–117.
136. Kazi H, Haddawy P, Suebnukarn S. Leveraging a domain ontology to increase the quality of feedback in an intelligent tutoring system. Lect Notes Comput Sci (including Subser Lect Notes Artif Intell Lect Notes Bioinformatics). 2010;6094 LNCS(PART 1):75–84.
137. Yau HT, Tsou LS, Tsai MJ. Octree-based Virtual Dental Training System with a Haptic Device. Comput Aided Des Appl. 2006;3(1–4):415–24

www.ingramcontent.com/pod-product-compliance
Ingram Content Group UK Ltd.
Pitfield, Milton Keynes, MK11 3LW, UK
UKHW021914190726
13853UKWH00002B/660